Asian Blepharoplasty and the Eyelid Crease

雙眼

Chinese Kanji characters for the word double eye, an abbreviated form for the term double eyelid crease

ふた
二
え
重
まぶた
瞼
じゅつ
術

Japanese words (consisting of both Kanji and Hiragana characters) describing the procedure for creation of a double eyelid crease

Asian Blepharoplasty and the Eyelid Crease

SECOND EDITION

William Pai-Dei Chen MD FACS

Clinical Professor of Ophthalmology
Department of Ophthalmology
University of California, Los Angeles, School of Medicine
Los Angeles, California, USA

Senior Attending Surgeon
Ophthalmic Plastic Surgery Service
Harbor-UCLA Medical Center
Torrance, California, USA

Private Practice
Long Beach and Newport Beach, California, USA
www.asianblepharoplasty.info
www.asianeyelid.com

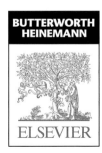

BUTTERWORTH
HEINEMANN

ELSEVIER

BUTTERWORTH
HEINEMANN
ELSEVIER

Butterworth–Heinemann is an affiliate of Elsevier Inc.

First edition 1995

ISBN-13: 978-0-7506-7574-1
ISBN-10: 0-7506-7574-8

British Library Cataloguing in Publication Data
A catalogue record for this book is available from the British Library

Library of Congress Cataloging in Publication Data
A catalog record for this book is available from the Library of Congress

Notice
Medical knowledge is constantly changing. Standard safety precautions must be followed, but as
new research and clinical experience broaden our knowledge, changes in treatment and drug therapy may become necessary or appropriate. Readers are advised to check the most current product
information provided by the manufacturer of each drug to be administered to verify the recommended
dose, the method and duration of administration, and contraindications. It is the responsibility of the
practitioner, relying on experience and knowledge of the patient, to determine dosages and the best
treatment for each individual patient. Neither the Publisher nor the author assume any liability for any
injury and/or damage to persons or property arising from this publication.

The Publisher

Printed in China
Last digit is the print number: 9   8   7   6   5   4   3   2   1

Commissioning Editor: Paul Fam
Development Editor: Claire Bonnett
Editorial Assistant: Amy Lewis
Project Manager: Gemma Lawson
Design Manager: Jayne Jones
Illustration Buyer: Gillian Murray
Illustrator: Gillian Lee
Marketing Manager(s) (UK/USA): Gaynor Jones/Lisa DaMico

With contributions from

Khoo Boo-Chai MD

Surgeon Director, Khoo Plastic Surgery Clinic, Singapore

Visiting Professor, Third Teaching Hospital, Department of Plastic Surgery

Beijing University, PR China

Visiting Professor, Shanghai Second Medical University

Ninth Hospital, Department of Plastic Surgery

Shanghai, PR China

Jung I. Park MD PhD FACS

Volunteer Clinical Assistant Professor, Department of Surgery

Indiana University Medical School, IN, USA

President, American Society of Asian Cosmetic Surgery

Dedication

To my parents Katie and Fred, my family, and my teachers

Contents

Preface

This is a comprehensive textbook exploring the art of creation of an eyelid crease in individual who may not have a crease or have an indistinct crease. When applied to patients of Asian ethnicity who do not have an eyelid crease, it is called 'Double eyelid surgery' in Asia and is the most popular cosmetic surgery there. The surgery and concepts appear deceptively simple, though in reality there is enough variables to make it one of the most demanding task when undertaken for aesthetic reasons.

This book is written in a progressive approach: the fundamentals is covered first, discussing terminology and the two main schools of techniques, as well as detailed discussion of the anatomy, before ascending to a more rigorous treatment of surgical techniques, pearls and pitfalls, personal observations, and finally to the more esoteric art of revisional surgery, covering evaluation, recognition of parameters and complications as well as more novel and original methods by this author to solve them. The readership is primarily aimed at practitioners and house officers in the fields of Plastic Surgery, Ophthalmolgy, Facial Plastic Surgery, Head and Neck surgery, Dermatology, as well as cosmetic surgeons in general who may be confronted with patients for this request. The materials are presented such that beginners, intermediate as well as advanced practitioners will all gain insights when an appropriate effort is expended in studying the book. Indeed one may find a different level of understanding as one go through and process the information at different turns.

In the twelve years since I completed the First Edition on 'Asian Blepharoplasty' in 1994, there has been continued refinement as well as worthy publications in this field. I realize that my techniques, as well as how I implement them have also evolved. The addition of new findings and publications as well as the evolution of my personal observations warrant an update on this vast topic. My purpose with the previous edition was to define the topic, its history, the general methods and techniques, as well as providing a solid foundation of terminology so that the topic can be discussed coherently and concisely. I did not want to get too esoteric in my first textbook since I was venturing into an area with conflicting ideas and terminology. The text was put together using a basic Macintosh SE desktop computer running Word program, using color slides and mostly black-and-white prints. Digital photography was not available then nor was digital printing. Since then the Internet has come to age and DVD technology is now available to make learning more visual and interactive.

The current Second Edition has twice the number of chapters (for a total of twenty) and three times the amount of text material, and includes a DVD. The color photos are all digital; the drawings are of a much finer quality and some are in color. The format of the book combines the style of a practical color atlas as well as a teaching manual, and is used in one of the author's recent text, 'Color Atlas of Cosmetic Oculofacial Surgery'. The images are arrayed such that the text on the page corresponds to them, and they are paired with comments including 'Pearls' and 'Pitfalls' when appropriate. Certain images have accompanying line drawings to clarify corresponding details. Detailed intraoperative findings are included in many of the clinical cases from the author's personal notebook. There are also quite a few more literature references included in the two comprehensive reference-spreadsheets, one covering the pioneering period between 1900 to 1950, and the other from mid-1950 to present. The book can be used as a learning text as well as a companion manual in an operating theater setting. I have tried to retain the simpler writing style and at all stages refrain from using complicated 'specialty-specific' terms, so that a general practitioner in this surgical field can read my material and assimilate the majority of my concepts. If I can achieve this, I am satisfied. Ironically I did not have any thoughts of working on a new edition until two separate house-officers who have worked with me in two different specialties complained to me that they can no longer purchase the now out-of-print First edition and that they can only find an occasional used copy on e-Bay selling for more than double the original sale price of a new copy. I am also encouraged by the interest shown in this field during my recent teaching trips to Korea and Hong Kong (China), as well as comments and encouragements from my colleagues from oversea.

This current project involved the use of a Macintosh G4 Powerbook, a Hewlett-Packard desktop computer, Sony digital editing software, Sony Digicam and DV recording, Nikon 950 and D-100 digital cameras, Sony T-1 and W-7 digital cameras, and Photoshop software for cropping purpose. Despite all these technical wizardry and tools available, the final determinant in surgical outcome still relates to correct concepts and application of meticulous techniques, as well as an open dialogue at all phases with each individual patient.

I wish to thank Dr. Kenichiro Kawai (at the Department of Plastic Surgery in Osaka University Graduate School of Medicine, Japan) and his colleagues (at the Keio University School of Medicine, and Hyogo College of Medicine, Hyogo, Japan) for graciously allowing me to include their anatomic finding of upper eyelid vascular arcades as well as the inclusion of stereoscopic angiograms. I am fortunate to have the participation and contribution from my friends Dr. Khoo Boo-Chai of Singapore and Dr. Jung Park of Indiana, each of whom contributed a chapter to this text. To them I express my sincere thanks.

Acknowledgements

I am grateful to the wonderful staff at Elsevier/Butterworth-Heinemann for their highly professional and competent support of this Second Edition of 'Asian Blepharoplasty and the Eyelid Crease'. This includes Paul Fam, Senior Editor who commissioned the project, Amy Lewis, Assistant Editor; Claire Bonnett (Developmental Editor), Lisa Damico (Marketing Manager), Megan Barth (Marketing Cordinator), and Colin McEwan (Digital Video Development), Gemma Lawson (Project Manager, Global Medicine and Surgery at Elsevier Ltd, Edinburgh) as well as graphic illustrators that have worked on the project. Their guidance and professional shepherding of this project is deeply appreciated.

I am blessed to have being under the guidance of Dr. Sonny McCord, Jr., my mentor during my fellowship training in Atlanta, Georgia.

Most of all I am very lucky to have the constant support of my wife Lydia and my children Katherine and Andrew.

William Pai-Dei Chen
2006

Introduction

Twenty years ago I was asked why I use the term *Asian blepharoplasty* rather than *oriental double eyelid procedure* when I lecture on the topic. I explained that, as a person who has been influenced by both eastern and western cultures, I believe that the term *oriental* is restrictive and does not adequately describe the diverse ethnic groups of the eastern hemisphere. I believe the term *Asian* is geographically more inclusive and representative of groups including Japanese, Chinese, Koreans, and southeast Asians. In particular, the term denotes people with Han ancestry, with the exception of Indians, Pakistanis, and Russians (although in the former Soviet Union many minorities have Mongolian or Han features, notably so in Kirgizstan).

Following similar reasoning, I believe that the operation necessary to construct an aesthetically pleasing upper eyelid crease requires reconstructive steps that involve the soft tissues anterior to the levator aponeurosis, namely skin, orbicularis oculi muscle, septum orbitale, and preaponeurotic fat pads. Anatomically, *blepharoplasty* is a more accurate term than either *double eyelid procedure* or *lid crease procedure*, which are more descriptive of the result than the procedure itself. With the evolution of surgical knowledge and a gradual diminution of stereotyping, *Asian blepharoplasty* has become the preferred term for describing the subtle details necessary to perform aesthetic procedures on the upper eyelids of Asian peoples.

There is an interesting difference and contradiction that I have observed from interacting with my Asian patients from around the world. Asians who have emigrated overseas or who are born and raised overseas tend to have a relatively ethnocentric view of themselves as a group and strive to retain some of their cultures and roots, to remain connected to their ancestry in much of their values and judgments, including the sense of body, health, and beauty. The native Asians (Chinese from China, Hong Kong, Taiwan and Asians from Korea, Japan, and Singapore) often will have a much more modern and westernized view of themselves when it comes to their sense of fashion and beauty, and may therefore be even more liberal than Asian-Americans or European-Asians. (An analogous situation can be noted: one can visit any of the Asian countries nowadays and observe the interior decor of recently established Asian restaurants versus those that are overseas and are still styled with an Asian theme, to see a large difference in their sense of modern interior decor. The Asian countries style is probably a good 10–20 years ahead of what is overseas.) We often think that native Asians are more conservative than overseas Asians when it comes to cosmetic surgery, but this is often not the case. By sheer numbers, there are far more Asian eyelid surgeries performed in Asia than there are here in the western hemisphere, averaging out population census: whether this results from socioeconomic wellbeing or the comparative costs of the procedure I am not sure.

There is also a far greater dichotomy of views with regard to the merits of cosmetic surgery in this country, perhaps because the United States is principally a free society. There are Asians who view cosmetic surgery as an integral and elective part of personal health, and there are others who view any form of cosmetic surgery or correction as a form of ethnic alteration. Once, long ago, I was invited as a 'Physician-Professor expert' to explain what Asian eyelid surgery is at an Asian Studies department at a major university in Los Angeles: I soon found myself receiving comments that this is a form of 'ethnic destruction' or stereotypical view of cultural dilution; and that this is akin to certain form of mutilation still practiced on women in some parts of the African continent. I am not a philosopher and I did not express any opinion then, though I find it odd that everything we do may be considered 'western'. As we arise in the morning (in western or modern Asian countries), we may take a shower or bath with western soap, brush with toothpaste, drink coffee, have a muffin, cereal or sandwich; put on a tie, shirt, belt and suit (or, if a woman, makeup, hair styling, western-style dresses and their handbags), get into our automobiles, buses, shuttles or subways – all western developments (not without first using the elevators!), and then go to work. We are then again surrounded by all kinds of western machinery, such as computers, cellular phones, facsimile machines, and great inventions such as the Internet and e-mail. Unless one does not perform any of above-mentioned chores, one certainly can remain a purist and live in a remote environment; and if so, then there is absolutely no need to do anything (not even going to a western-trained dentist to have your dental cavities fixed!).

As you read this book you will come across a myriad of different techniques, all trying to achieve the same goal. What should ultimately differentiate them should be the time-honoured objective determinants for the success of a surgical procedure, such as efficacy, or the ability to reach therapeutic goals, permanency, probability of morbidity and complications, and recurrence rate of the original condition. In blepharoplasty, this equates to achievement of an aesthetic goal, continuity and permanency, likelihood of asymmetry and complications, and rate of obliteration within a 3–5-year period. A practitioner is almost always driven by the force of demand in his community. For example, if patients are demanding a very low-set crease located in the midtarsal zone and are concerned about not having any skin incision, the suture ligation method is perfectly fine to use and achieves its goals well, provided the patients are well aware of the chance of subsequent disappearance of the crease, or minor irritations that may occur over the soft tissue of the eyelids if there were any permanent retained sutures (as used in most variants). If there is significant redundancy of pretarsal or preseptal tissues of the upper eyelid, the incisional blepharoplasty techniques are more applicable, provided they are carried out by a well qualified practitioner. It is therefore up to the practitioner and patient to come to a mutual understanding in terms of which method can achieve their goal, as well as being a sound procedure that can stand up to the test of time. Even this last statement can be debated, as you will certainly find patients and physicians (although a smaller pool) that may find the issue of permanency a matter of less relevant concern.

I am grateful to see that some of the terminology I used in the first edition of this book has filtered into general and acceptable use in the aesthetic and plastic surgery field, in publications, the media, as well as other surgeons' websites. An accurate description of surgical findings and techniques will improve the knowledge base for the whole field and ultimately benefit patient care.

William PD Chen

Historical Considerations

Chapter 1

William P.D. Chen

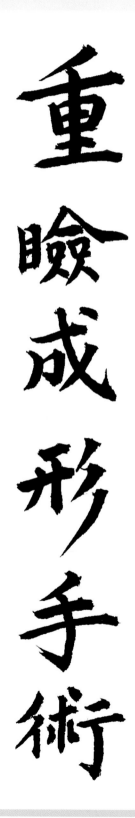

重瞼成形手術

Cosmetic Oculoplastic Surgery: Evolution of Double-Eyelid Cosmetic Surgery in the Japanese Literature

Publications in the early Japanese medical literature favored the suture ligation method. The first description of this method, by Mikamo,[1] was published in 1896 (see Appendix 1, and Appendix 2 under Shirakabe, 1985). Mikamo performed the procedure on a Japanese woman who did not have a crease in one of her upper eyelids. The crease was designed to be 6–8 mm from the ciliary margin. Three 4/0 braided silk sutures were used, passing through the full thickness of the lid from the conjunctiva to the outer layer of skin. The depth of the crease was adjusted by the number of days the sutures were left in, the range being 2–6 days.

As early as 1926, Uchida[2] described his suture ligation method for the double-eyelid operation. He performed the procedure on 1523 eyelids in 396 male and 444 female patients. Uchida described the crease configuration as a fan shape, that is, a somewhat rounded crease. The crease was designed to be 7–8 mm from the ciliary margin. Three buried catgut sutures were used on each lid, encompassing approximately 2 mm of eyelid tissue horizontally. The sutures were removed 4 days after placement.

The first mention of an external incision method dates to 1929, when Maruo[3] reported on both his suturing technique and his incision technique. Maruo's incision technique required a crease incision across the lid, designed to be 7 mm from the ciliary margin. The wound closure technique was a translid passage from the conjunctival side just above the superior tarsal border to the anterior skin surface. One 5/0 catgut suture was used to imbricate four throws along the superior tarsal border, attaching the skin edges to the underlying tarsal plate. The spacing between each throw of the stitch was about 5–6 mm. Maruo also discussed subcutaneous dissection 5 mm superior and inferior to the incision line.

In 1933, preference for a higher placement of the crease became evident when Hata[4] reported his suture ligation method. The crease line was placed 10 mm from the ciliary margin. Hata used three double-armed 5/0 braided silk sutures, passing them from tarsus to skin and fixing them to the skin surface using small beads. Each arm of the suture required 1-mm spacing for the bead to be tied. Stitches were removed after 8–10 days.

In a comprehensive and scholarly article in 1938, Hayashi[5] described the two methods of crease formation. His suture ligation technique was modeled after Mikamo's method but was novel in that it was designed for a nasally tapered crease. Three sutures were used on each lid. The central and lateral sutures were applied superior to the crease line or tarsal plate, whereas the medial suture was deliberately applied below the crease line or tarsal plate. Hayashi's incision method was also revolutionary, in that he advocated excision of the pretarsal orbicularis oculi muscle at the area of the incision. He also advocated the use of interrupted skin–tarsus–skin sutures, and in between skin–skin stitches consisting of 4/0 silk for wound closure. The crease was designed so that medially it was 5 mm from the ciliary margin, centrally 6 mm from the margin, and laterally 7 mm from the margin; in essence it was a nasally tapered crease. The sutures were removed after 4 days.

Inoue[6] in 1947 proposed dissecting the 'connective tissues' in the subcutaneous plane between the incision line and the ciliary margin. Sutures of 5/0 braided silk were used for skin–tarsus–skin closure; sutures were removed after only 2–3 days.

In 1950, Mitsui[7] continued the evolution of the double-eyelid crease procedure when he described the dissection and removal of pretarsal connective tissue, including pretarsal orbicularis muscle and pretarsal fat pads. Wound closure was carried out in two steps. First, five separate nylon sutures were used to stitch the inferior skin border to the anterior surface of the superior tarsal border and were tied individually. Second, 5/0 braided silk was used to close the incision site skin to skin. The nylon sutures were removed after 2–3 days, the silk sutures after 7–8 days.

Ohashi[8] described a double-eyelid crease operation using an electric coagulator. The cautery needle was applied vertically to the skin surface along the crease line until the skin blistered; two more rows of cauterization below the crease line followed. Hirose[9] and Ikegami[10] in 1951 briefly discussed incision methods but did not offer any new information.

The foregoing procedures were described only in the Japanese literature and were not readily available to western readers. As a result, the publication of articles on this procedure in western medical journals in the 1950s made the procedure seem new (and western) in concept. Between 1896 and 1950, 11 articles relating to the suture ligation methods and eight articles on external incision methods were published in the Japanese medical literature (see Appendix I).

Much of the later western literature on this subject described techniques quite similar to those described in the early Japanese publications (see Chapters 5 and 6 for a continuation of historical publications from the 1950s onward).

References

1. Mikamo K. A technique in the double eyelid operation. J Chugaishinpo 1896.
2. Uchida K. The Uchida method for the double-eyelid operation in 1,523 cases. Jpn J Ophthalmol 1926;30:593.
3. Maruo M. Plastic construction of a 'double-eyelid.' Jpn Rev Clin Ophthalmol 1929;24:393–406.
4. Hata B. Application of eyelid clamp and beads in 'double-eyelid' operation. Jpn Rev Clin Ophthalmol 1933;28:491–494.
5. Hayashi K. The double eyelid operation. Jpn Rev Clin Ophthalmol 1938;33:1000–1010, 1098–1110.
6. Inoue S. The double eyelid operation. Jpn Rev Clin Ophthalmol 1947;27:306.
7. Mitsui Y. Plastic reconstruction of a double eyelid. Jpn Rev Clin Ophthalmol 1950;44:19.
8. Ohashi K. The double eyelid operation using electrocautery. Jpn Rev Clin Ophthalmol 1951;46:723.
9. Hirose K. The double eyelid operation. Jpn Rev Clin Ophthalmol 1950;45:374.
10. Ikegami T. Brief discussion on the double eyelid operation. Jpn Rev Clin Ophthalmol 1951;46:706–707.

Comparative Anatomy of the Eyelids Chapter 2

William P.D. Chen

The Upper Lid and Crease

Studies have shown that about 50% of Asians do not have an upper eyelid crease; the other 50% have at least some form of crease. Eyes without a lid crease are described as having a 'single eyelid' (Fig. 2-1), whereas those with two segments of lid between the eyebrow and the eyelashes have 'double eyelids' (Fig. 2-2). Most of the plastic surgery literature of the 1950s[1,2] was based on the assumption that all Asians are without an eyelid crease and that all Caucasians have an upper lid crease.

Asians born with a crease appear to have a wider palpebral fissure and larger eyes and are culturally perceived to be more alert and friendly than those with a single eyelid (Fig. 2-3). The cultural ideal of feminine beauty also influences the desire for a double eyelid: having a double eyelid allows greater latitude in the application of cosmetics to make the eyes and face more aesthetically pleasing. It is therefore understandable that some women without a crease may wish for one, provided the means are available.

To some westerners who presume that all Asians are without a crease, such an endeavor equates to 'westernization' or 'occidentalization.' In the author's opinion, however, it merely equates to an attempt to look like their fellow Asians who do have a crease over their upper eyelids.[3]

The growing popularity of Asian blepharoplasty has been incorrectly interpreted as resulting from the influence of western culture after World War II and the Korean war, a manifestation of which was believed to be a desire on the part of Asians to blend in with Caucasians, to look westernized or occidental. The author has had the opportunity to travel extensively and to teach in Asia. It is my perception that the idea of beauty transcends time, geographic boundaries, and ethnicity. I have found that the increasing number of patients undergoing Asian blepharoplasty has more to do with an increasing awareness that such procedures are available than with the cultural influence of the west. Clinical experience teaches that Asians do not want to look Caucasian. A frequent postoperative complaint is that the procedure results in a semilunar crease, a feature that, although characteristic of Caucasians, is aesthetically displeasing in Asians.[4]

The essential differences in the upper eyelid structure between Caucasians and Asians have been studied in cadaver samples by Doxanas[5] and Jeong et al.[6] The fundamental difference between the subset of those Asian eyelids without a crease and a Caucasian eyelid which possesses a crease appears to be the lower point of fusion of the orbital septum on to the levator aponeurosis in Asians.

Individuals with a Lid Crease

In Caucasians who have a crease[5] (Fig. 2-4) the orbital septum fuses with the levator aponeurosis approximately 5–10 mm above the superior tarsal border. Below this point, the terminal interdigitations of the levator aponeurosis insert towards the subdermal surface of the pretarsal and preseptal upper lid skin, with maximal concentration along the superior tarsal border and spreading inferiorly.[7] Collin[8] has detailed electron microscopic findings of fusion of the terminal fibers of the levator aponeurosis with the septae that are in between the pretarsal and preseptal orbicularis muscle fibers; he was unable to show any direct attachment to the skin in that particular study.

There has been a subsequent study in China using scanning electron microscopy that described the presence of aponeurotic fibers penetrating the orbicularis fibers to fuse with the skin underneath a crease. In this study published in 2001, Cheng and Xu[9] reported using scanning electron microscopy and detecting bunched fibers of levator aponeurosis penetrating through the orbicularis muscle and fusing with the skin on the area of the eyelid crease in those patients born with a crease, versus those without. These differences were not detectable using conventional light microscopy. The authors described the arrangement of

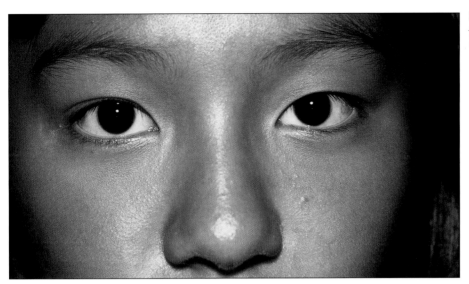

Fig. 2-1 Partially shielded crease over the right upper lid. Absent crease or 'single eyelid' over left upper lid.

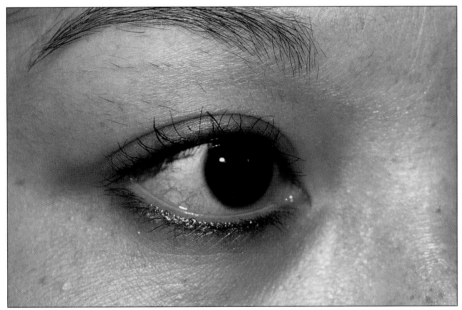

Fig. 2-2 Double eyelid. Parallel crease configuration.

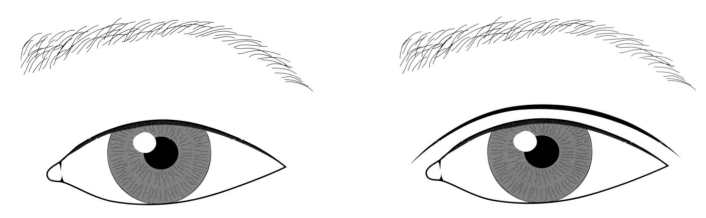

A

B

Fig. 2-3 Left palpebral fissure. **(A)** Without crease. **(B)** With crease. The crease gives the impression of a larger eye opening.

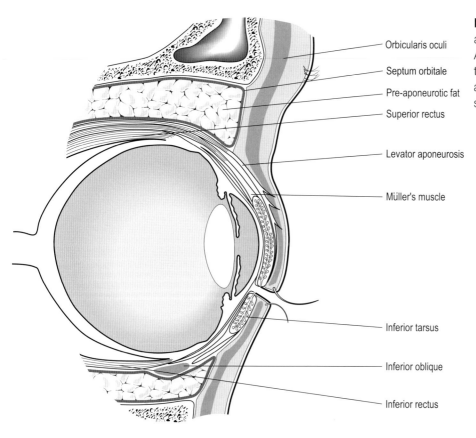

Fig. 2-4 A typical Caucasian eyelid with a natural upper eyelid crease. Aponeurotic fibers form interdigitations to the pretarsal orbicularis oculi muscle and a subdermal attachment along the superior tarsal border.

Orbicularis oculi

Septum orbitale

Pre-aponeurotic fat

Superior rectus

Levator aponeurosis

Müller's muscle

Inferior tarsus

Inferior oblique

Inferior rectus

these bundled fibers as being different from that of the fibers in the intermuscular septum. The bundles were thinner, unidirectional, and aligned as threads. They noted that where these fibers pass through the orbicularis to attach to the subcutaneous fibers they were linear in shape, closely aligned and clearly visualized, whereas the fibers of the intermuscular septum were thicker and aligned in a disorderly fashion. Of interest is the observation that in those eyelids with a crease the orbicularis bundles lying transversely were arrayed sparsely and loosely in a single layer, in contrast to those in a single eyelid (i.e. without a crease), which had muscle tissues that were dense and muscle bundles arrayed in a stratified manner. Their overall conclusion is that a fiber link between levator aponeurosis and the upper eyelid skin results in the formation of the palpebral sulcus (crease) in the double eyelid. They draw the inference that the purpose of most double-eyelid procedures should be to establish a stable attachment between levator aponeurosis and the eyelid skin. They further stated that the obstructing effect of the orbicularis in single-lidded individual could explain why the surgical outcome is unpredictable with the suturing

method. Using the incision method, the excision of a suitable amount of orbicularis muscle changes the dynamics of the upper eyelid and assures a good aesthetic outcome. The authors recommended the incision method with supratarsal fixation in order to establish a stable attachment between the levator aponeurosis and the eyelid skin.

A similar study published in the same year by Morikawa et al.[10] described the scanning electron microscopic findings in single- versus double-eyelid samples taken from Japanese cadaver specimens. They were able to trace the collagen fibers that branched off from the levator aponeurosis, running through the orbicularis oculi muscle layer and inserting at the subcutaneous layer just within the crease space indentation. These fibers do not contact the skin directly, but become continuous with the collagen fibers in the subcutaneous tissues.

Hwang et al.[11] attempted to show that the orbital septum consists of an outer (whitish, superficial) layer and an inner layer which, upon meeting the levator aponeurosis inferiorly, then reflects superiorly and continues with the sheath of the levator muscle, which they

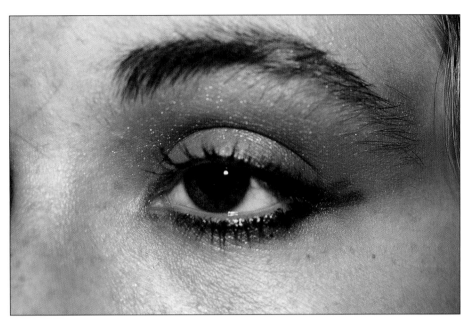

Fig. 2-5 Caucasian upper lid creases that are high and semilunar in shape.

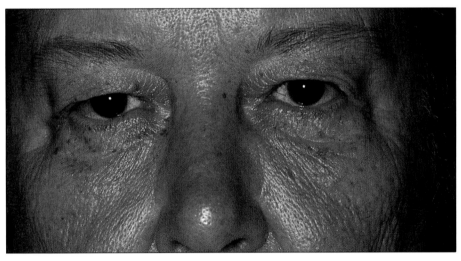

Fig. 2-6 Elderly Caucasian patient before blepharoplasty. Redundant preaponeurotic fat pads and dermatochalasis of the upper lid form a hood over the previously distinctive crease.

termed levator sheath. There were several line drawings in their article attempting to illustrate this concept, and a light microscopic slide that showed what purported to be the inner layer of the orbital septum and the sheath of the levator, but the higher-magnification slide did not have a portion showing that one continues into the other, which was their premise. There had been previous description of the anterior lining of the levator (levator sheath) descending and then reflecting up the back surface of the orbital septum to reach the superior orbital rim,[12] but there had been no concrete study illustrating that the reverse is true, i.e. that the orbital septum has two layers, a posterior layer that actually reflects back on to the levator surface to form its sheath. The authors further postulate that the reason for some crease procedures failing to form a crease is due to the presence of remnants of the inner layer of the orbital septum on the aponeurotic surface, which may have been attached to skin surgically instead of the desired skin–aponeurosis attachment. They also stated that there may be remnants of fat behind this fourth layer, the inner layer of the orbital septum lying on the anterior surface of the aponeurosis, and the underlying levator aponeurosis, and that these need to be reflected away before carrying out the skin–aponeurosis fixation.

Bang et al.[13] argued against the conventional theory that the levator termination inserts into the skin to form the crease. The authors proposed that this theory is more accurate, i.e. that the absence of a crease is associated with a lower position of the septum in a single eyelid without a crease, hence there is more inferiorly migrated fat and the eyelid is thicker than one that has a crease, which is thinner and has a tighter pretarsal skin zone. The crease in this theory corresponds to the lowermost edge of the orbital fat, or the lower level of the orbital septum, which is usually 2–3 mm above the highest point of insertion of the levator aponeurosis. In an excellent brief discussion following the above-mentioned paper by Bang et al., Boo-Chai[14] stated that below the lowermost edge of the orbital fat there are fine filamentous condensations of the connective tissue that connect the aponeurosis to the connective tissue septa between the fibers of the orbicularis oculi muscles. The crease lies in the pretarsal skin at the superior insertion of these fibers and serves as a useful external landmark of the common boundary between the lowermost edge of the orbital fat and the filamentous connective tissue condensation fibers. When the eye opens, the pull of the levator is transmitted via these fibers to the pretarsal skin–muscle complex. The pretarsal skin below the crease moves as a single unit upward and backward, like the visor of a helmet. The orbital fat moves back into the orbit, and the superior palpebral fold is formed by the lid skin scrolling down at the upper lid crease. Boo-Chai further observed that the pretarsal skin is soft and very thin, with little space between the dermis and the subcutaneous areolar plane to the orbicularis beneath. The skin above the upper lid crease is comparatively thick, with some subcutaneous fat, with the crease lying at the junction of this region. He favored the continued use of the term levator expansion (extension).

The Fat Pads of the Upper Lids

In terms of fat distribution and compartments, Uchida[15] described the presence of four areas of fat pads in Asian upper eyelids. He described the subcutaneous fat, the pretarsal fat, the 'central' (submuscular or preseptal) fat pads and the 'orbital' fat pad, which is now better known as the preaponeurotic fat pad (see Fig. 2-7).

Miyake et al.[16] described upper eyelid MRI findings in those with a crease versus those without. He observed that the 'orbital fat' normally returns into the orbit as the upper eyelid opens in someone with a crease, but that when the fat does not return then crease formation is prevented. He correctly observed that the crease folds in at the junction between the thin skin without subcutaneous fat (pretarsal area) and the thick skin with subcutaneous fat (preseptal area).

The preaponeurotic fat pad is limited in its inferiormost position by the junction (or reflection) of the septum with the levator aponeurosis and does not tend to interfere with the terminal insertions of the aponeurotic fibers. When the levator contracts and pulls the tarsal plate up, the lid forms a crease just above the superior tarsal border, with the skin superior to the crease forming the fold (Fig. 2-5). The rigidity of the upper tarsus and the firm adherence of the skin over the pretarsal region effectively results in a pretarsal platform vectoring superoposteriorly underneath the overhanging fold of skin and the preaponeurotic tissue platform. In elderly people there is frequently a lack of preaponeurotic fat pads and the presence of dermatochalasis causing hooding over the previously distinctive lid crease (Fig. 2-6).

In those Asians who do not have a lid crease (Fig. 2-7) the anatomic studies of Doxanas[5] and Anderson[7] appeared to confirm that they have a lower point of attachment of the orbital septum to the levator aponeurosis, frequently as low as the superior tarsal border. The author has seen patients whose orbital septum fuses with the upper tarsus below the superior tarsal border, halfway down its anterior surface (Fig. 2-8). This lower point of fusion permits the presence of the preaponeurotic fat pad at a lower point on the aponeurosis, giving the eyelid a fuller appearance. The lower preaponeurotic fat pad may in turn prevent the attachment of the terminal interdigitations of the levator aponeurosis along the superior tarsal border to the pretarsal orbicularis oculi muscle fibers.

Subcutaneous fat, sub-brow (submuscular, suborbicularis, or preseptal) fat and pretarsal fat infiltration as described by Uchida[15] may be seen. The presence of pretarsal fat pads may also disrupt the terminal interdigitations of the aponeurosis, if we are to presume that Collin's[8] and Cheng's[9] scanning electron microscopy findings are accurate and applicable to those Asian eyelids without a crease. The clinical picture is a puffy

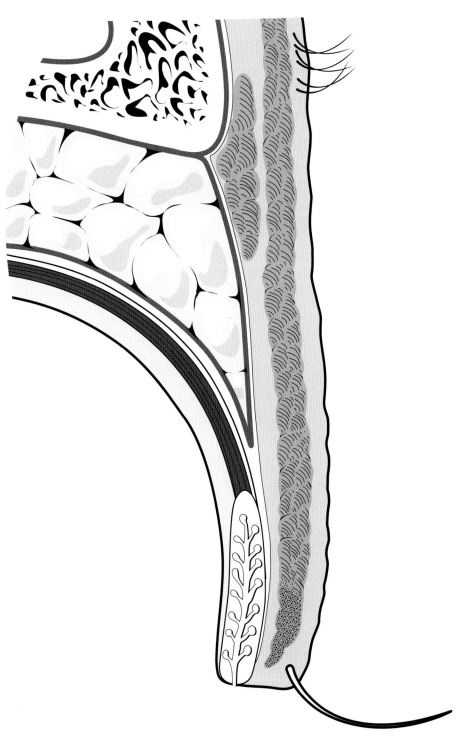

Fig. 2-7 Asian upper eyelid without a crease. Note the absence of terminal interdigitations of the levator aponeurosis and the relatively lower point of fusion of the orbital septum.

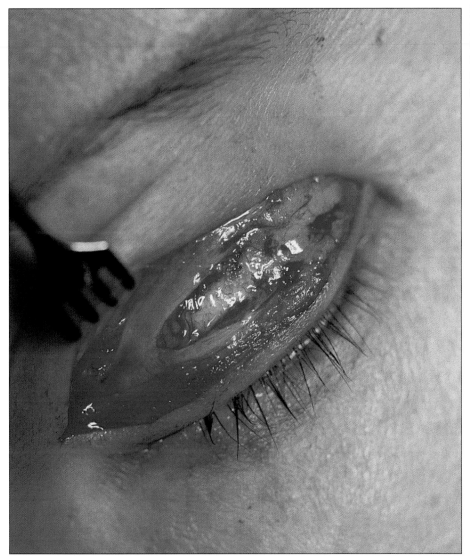

Fig. 2-8 Right upper lid with a very low point of fusion of the orbital septum along the anterior surface of the upper tarsus. Preaponeurotic fat can be seen posterior to the surgically opened septum.

'single eyelid' without a crease (Fig. 2-9). With age, the interval change in Caucasians tends to be an increase in prominence of the preaponeurotic and nasal fat pads as they migrate forward and inferiorly. The elderly Asian eyelid tends to simply manifest more skin redundancy, as the lid has always been comparatively full owing to the lower position of the preaponeurotic fat and fascial tissues (Fig. 2-10). Some degree of gravitational inward settling of the orbital fat in the upper half of the orbital space does occur with aging, therefore the volume of fat seen clinically over the upper eyelid may be variable.

An intriguing hypothetical explanation for Collin's and Cheng's finding that in upper eyelids with a crease there are interdigitations of the terminal aponeurotic fibers to septae[8] among the pretarsal and preseptal orbicularis muscle, or insertion[9] into the subcutaneous area of the crease, giving a firm pretarsal platform to 'telescope' back to form a crease, is that in those Asians who have only a rudimentary crease it is not obvious, owing to the presence of pretarsal fat pads in the pretarsal orbicularis muscles (Fig. 2-11). The presence of these fine fat pads may dilute the effect of the aponeurotic fiber interdigitations among the pretarsal orbicularis fibers, creating a puffier and less rigid pretarsal platform, and in conjunction with the inferior migration of the orbital septum and preaponeurotic fat pads it produces a full lid with no opportunity for the clear demarcation of a crease. A corollary to this would be that in those Asians who do have a crease, there is a

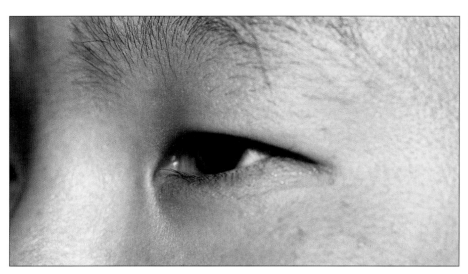

Fig. 2-9 Single eyelid with upper eyelid hooding.

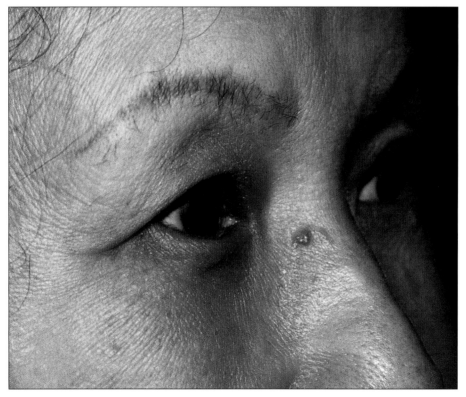

Fig. 2-10 Elderly Asian before blepharoplasty. The patient has redundant dermatochalasis rather than an active prolapse of preaponeurotic fat pads.

paucity of pretarsal fat pads: the terminal fibers from the aponeurosis interdigitate with the pretarsal orbicularis muscle as before, and they still have a rigid pretarsal platform to form a crease, even though their preaponeurotic fat pads are at a lower level than in Caucasians. Caucasians who previously had a crease may lose it with age, as the pretarsal platform loses its rigidity owing to dehiscence of the orbicularis fibers and infiltration of fat into that area (see Fig. 2-6). In both Asians and Caucasians who do not have a crease it is possible to create one by placing sutures that attach the skin to the levator aponeurosis. Excessive pretarsal dissection and debulking can lead to multiple crease formation (Fig. 2-12).

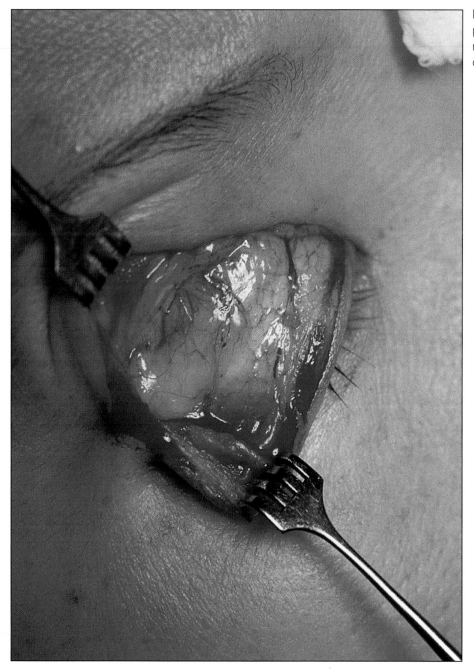

Fig. 2-11 The presence of pretarsal fat pads within pretarsal orbicularis oculi muscle in an Asian upper lid without a crease.

Yoo[17] formed a crease simply by trimming the pretarsal fat and placing 'basting' sutures. This procedure eliminated the dead space formed by the removal of pretarsal tissues but did not involve direct stitch attachment of the levator aponeurosis or tarsal plate. The net result was a rigid pretarsal platform that allowed crease formation. It is highly unlikely, however, that there would be no aponeurotic adhesions to the pretarsal tissues after such a maneuver.

The Medial Canthus

According to Johnson,[18] the epicanthal folds can be divided into at least four clinical types: epicanthus supraciliaris, epicanthus palpebralis, epicanthus tarsalis, and epicanthus inversus. Epicanthus supraciliaris is very uncommon. It originates from the brow and curves down towards the lacrimal sac (Fig. 2-13). Epicanthus palpebralis rises above the upper tarsus and

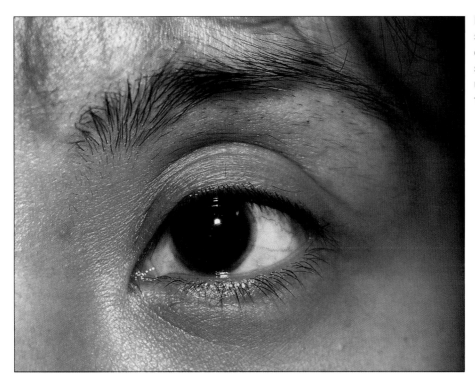

Fig. 2-12 Multiple creases and a hollow supratarsal sulcus secondary to excessive dissection in the pretarsal and supratarsal space. The patient has undergone a lid crease procedure through an anterior approach.

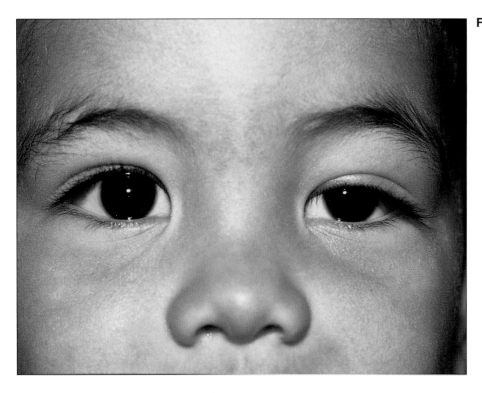

Fig. 2-13 Mild epicanthus supraciliaris.

extends to the inferior orbital rim (Fig. 2-14). Epicanthus tarsalis rises from the upper lid crease and merges into the skin near the medial canthus (Fig. 2-15). Johnson called this configuration 'Mongolian eye'. In epicanthus inversus, the fold rises from the lower lid and extends to the upper lid over the medial canthus (Fig. 2-16).

Of the four types of epicanthus described by Johnson,[18] Asians usually have epicanthus tarsalis. This configuration is a subtle fold of skin that arises from

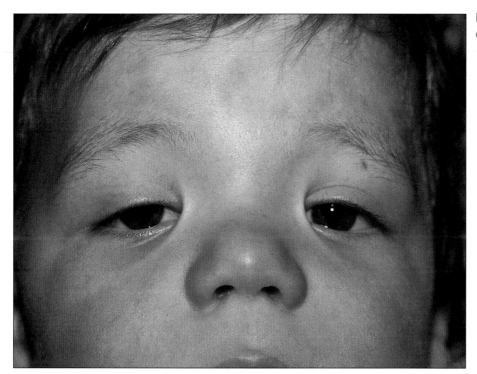

Fig. 2-14 Two-year-old Eurasian with epicanthus palpebralis.

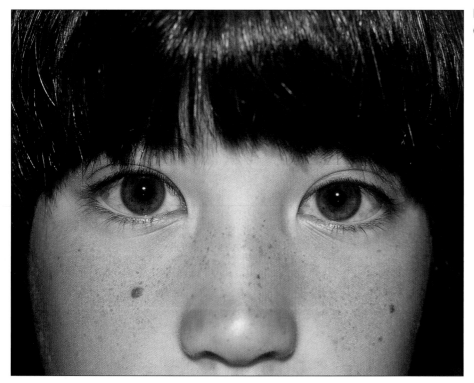

Fig. 2-15 Six-year-old Eurasian with epicanthus tarsalis.

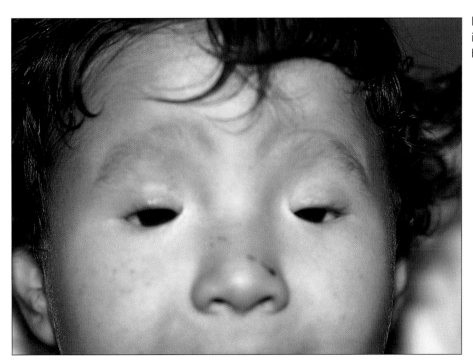

Fig. 2-16 Child with epicanthus inversus, part of the congenital blepharophimosis syndrome.

the medial canthal angle and courses laterally, forming a small medial upper lid fold, toward a point between the medial third and the medial half of the upper lid. Some Asian children may appear to have an epicanthus palpebralis (Fig. 2-17A,B), in which the fold covers the upper and lower lids equally across the medial canthus. With growth and development, however, the fold appears to be transformed into a medial upper lid fold. This may be the result of the development of the nasal bridge (Fig. 2-18). The medial upper lid fold is often seen in patients who already have a natural crease (Fig. 2-19).

Most articles[19–21] in the literature seem to focus on the correction of epicanthus palpebralis and epicanthus inversus. The latter is a condition more often associated with the syndrome of congenital blepharophimosis. Most repairs are a variation of the double-Z or Y-V-plasty. These techniques are ill-suited to the correction of the medial upper lid fold in Asians.

The author[3,4,22,23] tends to be conservative in the correction of these medial upper lid folds, for the following reasons. First, it is hard to call something pathologic when it occurs naturally in a large percentage of the population, considering that there are at least two to three billion Asians living on this planet. Second, Asians tend to have thicker skin near the nasal bridge, which is more reactive and prone to hyper-

trophic scarring in the thick medial canthal skin area. Third, a medially tapered crease that merges with the origin of a mild medial upper lid fold or 'epicanthus tarsalis' provides an aesthetically natural crease, as seen in those Asians who do have a lid crease. Fourth, the fold often evolves and regresses as the individual reaches adulthood. These small medial canthal folds are almost always a very small version of a true epicanthus and do not warrant being labeled with a term implying pathologic status.

Upper Tarsus

Asians tend to be smaller built than Caucasians. Their upper tarsus is often only 6.5–8.5 mm in vertical dimension compared to Caucasians,[22,23] in whom the average is 10 mm, ranging from 9.5 mm upwards.

Vascular Supply of the Upper Eyelid

Kawai et al.[24] studied the upper eyelids in seven fresh cadaver specimens, presumably of Asian origin. The specimens were systemically injected with a lead oxide–gelatin mixture and stereoscopic radiographic records of the anastomotic vessels were made, followed by macroscopic dissection. The authors found four

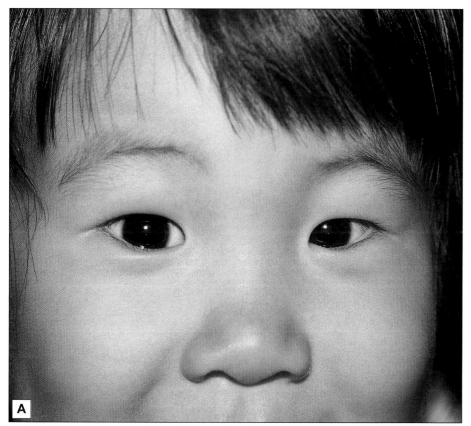

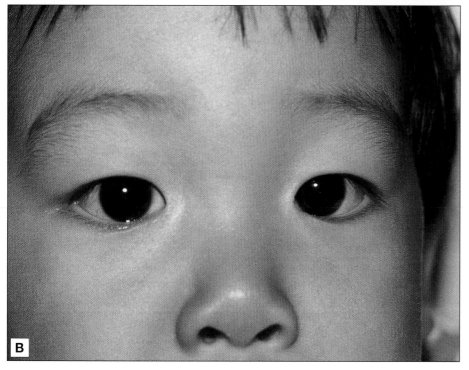

Fig. 2-17 (A) A 3-year-old child and **(B)** a 1-year-old child with slight epicanthal fold (a more appropriate term would be medial upper lid fold). The presence of this fold in Asian children frequently makes them appear to have esotropia (inward turning of the visual axis).

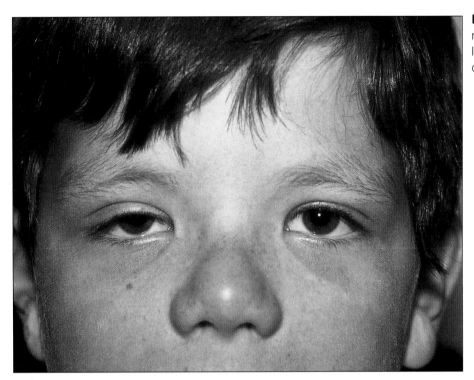

Fig. 2-18 Same child as in Figure 2-14, now 6 years of age and showing much less of the epicanthus palpebralis, with development of the nasal bridge.

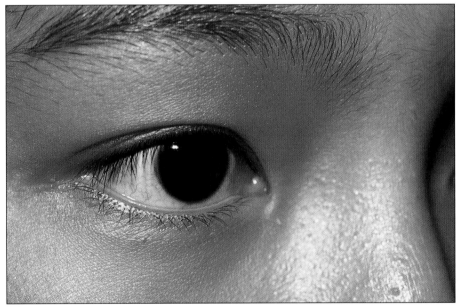

Fig. 2-19 Medial upper lid fold in an Asian teenager born with a nasally tapered crease.

main arterial arcades in the upper eyelids, i.e. marginal, peripheral, superficial orbital and deep orbital. They described vertical branches arising from each arcade, with the vertical branches of the superficial orbital arcade lying anterior to the preseptal orbicularis, the vertical branches of the deep orbital arcade behind the same orbicularis, and the vertical branches between the marginal and peripheral arcades lying both in front of and beneath the upper tarsal plate (Fig. 2-20).

The marginal and peripheral arcades were formed by the anastomosis of the medial and lateral palpebral arteries, which were branches of the ophthalmic and lacrimal arteries. The marginal arcade was situated between the orbicularis and the tarsal plate; it lay just

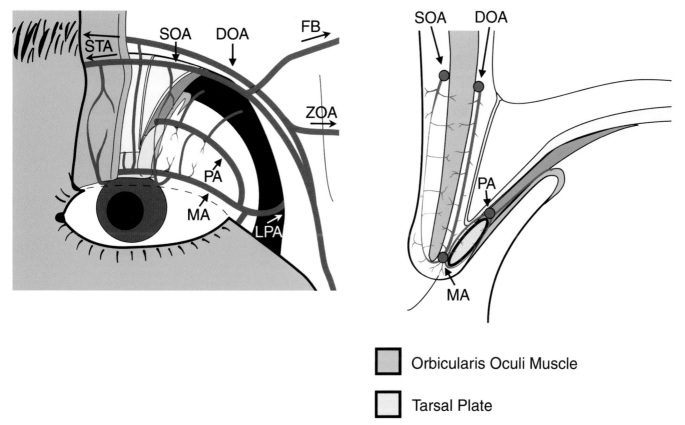

Orbicularis Oculi Muscle

Tarsal Plate

Fig. 2-20 There are four arterial arcades in the upper eyelid: the marginal arcade (MA), the peripheral arcade (PA), the superficial orbital arcade (SOA), and the deep orbital arcade (DOA). Each provides small vertical branches running on both sides of the orbicularis oculi muscle or on both sides of the tarsal plate. From these small vertical branches, fine vessels branch off to the skin, muscle, and tarsal plate. FB, frontal branch of the superficial temporal artery; ZOA, zygomatico-orbital artery; LPA, lateral palpebral artery; STA, supratrochlear artery. (Reproduced with permission from Kawai et al[24], Journal of Plastic and Reconstructive Surgery. Lippincott, Williams and Wilkins.)

anterior to the lower margin of the tarsal plate and gave off small vertical branches that ascended tortuously on both sides of the orbicularis and on both sides of the tarsal plate. These branches provided fine vessels to the skin, muscle, and tarsal plate. In addition to these small vertical branches, the marginal arcades provided fine vessels to the free edge of the upper lid. The peripheral arcade coursed in Müller's muscle along the superior tarsal border, and gave off vertical branches that descended on both sides of the tarsal plate. The descending branches (of the peripheral arcade) running over the tarsal plate anastomosed with the ascending branches arising from the marginal arcade, whereas the descending branches running beneath the tarsus separated into fine vessels and formed a vascular plexus with the ascending branches arising from the marginal arcade (Fig. 2-21).

The superficial and deep orbital arcades were formed by the anastomosis of the branches of the zygomatico-orbital artery, the transverse facial artery, or the frontal branch of the superficial temporal artery laterally and the branches of the supratrochlear artery, the ophthalmic artery, or the medial palpebral artery medially. Of these, the supratrochlear artery contributed significantly to both the superficial and deep orbital arcades, the latter running along the superior orbital rim. The terms superficial and deep refer to the level of the preseptal orbicularis oculi layer. Both the superficial and deep orbital arcades gave off vertical branches that descended anterior and posterior to the orbicularis and anastomosed with ascending branches from the marginal arcade. The authors further noted that the vertical vessels running over the orbicularis oculi traversed obliquely (connecting the marginal to

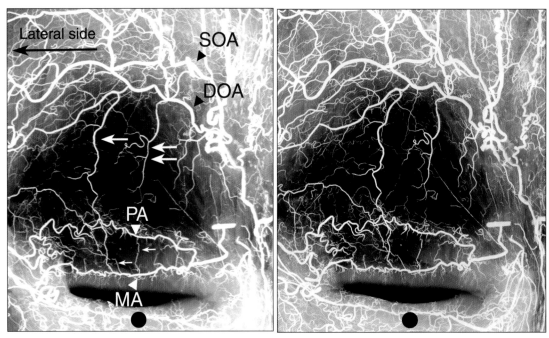

Fig. 2-21 Stereoscopic radiographic angiograms of the right upper lid. To superimpose the images of the left and right black dots, the reader should cross (converge) their eyes and then elevate their gaze towards the center of the paired images, which for someone with binocular vision will then yield a stereoscopic view. It should be observed that each arcade branches off the small vertical vessels (large and small arrows), and that the vertical vessels from the marginal arcade (MA) anastomoses with the vertical vessels from the other three arcades.

Large single arrow, vertical vessel connecting the marginal arcade and the deep orbital arcade (DOA); large double arrows, vertical vessel connecting the marginal arcade and the superficial orbital arcade (SOA); small arrows, vertical vessels connecting the marginal arcade and the peripheral arcade (PA). (Reproduced with permission from Kawai et al[24], Journal of Plastic and Reconstructive Surgery. Lippincott, Williams and Wilkins.)

the superficial arcade) rather than vertically, as with those that ran under the orbicularis, which connected the deep orbital arcade to the marginal arcade. They did not observe any single dominant intramuscular vessel within the orbicularis and deduced that its blood supply must therefore come from the fine vessels from the vertical branches. The authors implied that their method of study provided an undistorted assessment of the arterial structure of the upper eyelid.

Kim et al.[25] reported an incidence of 25 among 230 eyelids where an artery thought to be a variation of the lacrimal artery was found superficial to the orbital septum and inferolateral to the levator muscle, at a location 4–5 mm medial from the lateral canthus. After piercing the levator it was observed to connect with the lateral palpebral artery behind the levator muscle. This lateral vessel was nicked in 14 cases and the bleeding arterial end retracted posteriorly behind the levator to form a hematoma in the postaponeurotic space. This resulted in swelling, secondary ptosis, and difficulty in designing the lateral portion of the eyelid crease. Clamping the bleeding vessel was noted to be more effective than electrocautery when this occurred. Besides postulating that this might be a variant of a branch of the lacrimal artery, the authors also mentioned the possibility of a communicating artery between the peripheral arcade and the marginal arcade, or that this might be a medially displaced lacrimal artery. They mentioned that a cadaver dissection with latex injected into the ophthalmic artery was in progress.

In a somewhat similar study, Hwang et al.[26] described the occasional presence of a laterally located artery, named the lateral septoaponeurotic artery (LaSA), as a branch of the superior lateral palpebral artery after it divides into the peripheral arcade, the

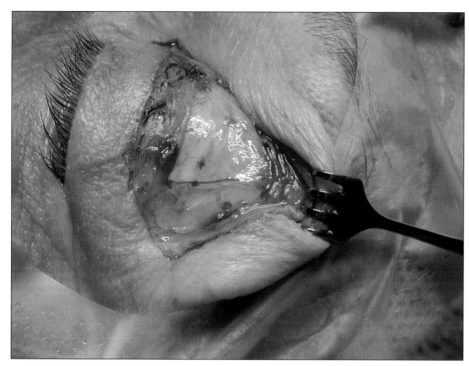

Fig. 2-22 Lateral septoaponeurotic artery found on the left upper eyelid during blepharoplasty: the skin–orbicularis layer had been peeled off after incision on the upper and lower skin edges using Ellmann's radiofrequency unit. (Image courtesy of WPD Chen.)

other being the marginal arcade. It was detected in 50 eyelids (11%) out of 460 operated on. (The superior lateral palpebral artery is a branch of the lacrimal artery, itself a branch of the ophthalmic artery.) The LaSA arises from the superior portion of the peripheral arcade, which runs along the superior tarsal border. From the peripheral arcade it pierces the levator aponeurosis and orbital septum at the upper level of the tarsal plate and is seen coursing on the surface of the orbital septum, about 5 mm inside the lateral canthus (Fig. 2-22). It anastomoses with a branch of the supraorbital artery at the superior aspect of the orbit. The authors commented that care should be taken in incising the lateral aspect of the septum, as severance of the LaSA may cause severe bleeding, hematoma formation and temporary ptosis, as well as retraction of the bleeding point and the formation of hematoma in the postaponeurotic plane. This may occur during use of the incisional method as well as the stitch method, which involves the placement of stitches over the lateral portion of the upper eyelid. This makes the surgeon's task of following his designed crease difficult. The authors recommended specific visual examination of the lateral aspect of the orbital septum prior to any horizontal transection.

Hematoma may also occur separately following injury to the perforating branch of the marginal arcade:

there is occasionally a larger branch of the arcade running perpendicularly upward and piercing the aponeurosis near its insertion on the anterior surface of the upper tarsus, where it may be injured when the lower incisional skin edge is manipulated during surgery. This, however, is separate from the LaSA.

Facial Anatomy

Onizuka and Iwanami[27] noted that the Japanese characteristically have a flat face, a mesocephalic head shape, and eyes that are not as deeply recessed in the orbit as in Caucasians. They noted that the lateral canthus is often 10° superior to the medial canthus. To produce an aesthetically pleasing result, they made an upper lid crease and removed any upper lid hooding to make the palpebral fissure appear wider and more open. Although the author does not believe that most Asians have a lateral canthus 10° above the medial canthus, some of Onizuka and Iwanami's observations may be correct.

Concept of Facial Symmetry

Song,[28] in 1988, wrote that since ancient times Chinese portrait artists have followed the rule of 'horizontal

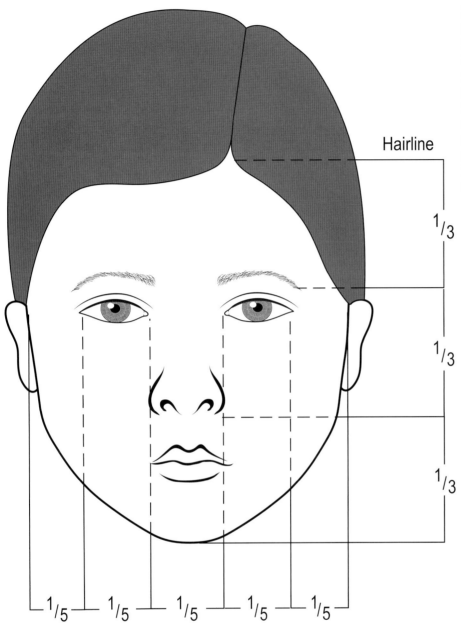

Hairline

$1/3$

$1/3$

$1/3$

$1/5$ $1/5$ $1/5$ $1/5$ $1/5$

Fig. 2-23 Rule of horizontal thirds and vertical fifths. The symmetric thirds are the distances from the hairline to the brow, from the brow to the base of the nose, and from the base of the nose to the chin. The fifths are the distances from the auditory canal to the lateral canthus, from the lateral canthus to the medial canthus, from medial canthus to medial canthus, from medial canthus to lateral canthus, and from lateral canthus to external auditory canal.

thirds, vertical fifths' when portraying the ideal face (Fig. 2-23). The symmetric thirds are the distances from the hairline to the brow, from the brow to the base of the nose, and from the base of the nose to the chin. The vertical fifths are identical to the western concept of the rule of fifths: the distance from the auditory canal to the lateral canthus, from the lateral canthus to the medial canthus, from medial canthus to the opposite medial canthus, from medial canthus to lateral canthus, and from lateral canthus to external auditory canal. An ideal palpebral fissure should be equal to one-fifth the width of the face. Interestingly, most patients with a single eyelid who desire a lid crease tend to have a palpebral fissure that is narrower than the ideal (Fig. 2-24); their eyes appear inharmonious with the rest of the face.

In attempting to match eyelid and crease configuration to the facial configuration, Song also mentioned six facial shapes and the eight factors that influence a crease. The six possible facial shapes seen in the average Asian population include square, rectangular, round, oval, triangular (with the base down), and diamond.

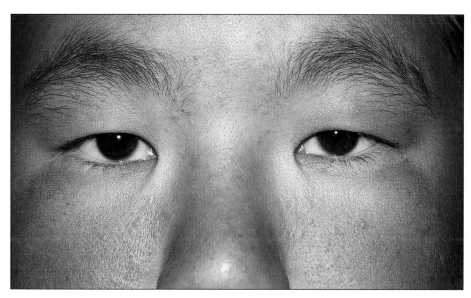

Fig. 2-24 Asian patient before Asian blepharoplasty. Note that the width of the palpebral fissure appears to be less than the intercanthal distance or the distance from the lateral canthus to the ear canal.

The eight factors that influence a crease are really the three variants of crease height (broad, average and narrow) and the five combinations of crease shape.

1. Parallel crease, favored by Song for a person with a stable temperament and a mild personality, a cheerful and happy person.
2. Medially narrow (<7–8 mm) and laterally broad crease (7–10 mm). Used for a person with a rectangular, stern face, a serious person.
3. Laterally narrow and medially broad crease. The eyelid appears hooded down laterally, producing a sad face and a triangular eye configuration. Not recommended.
4. Broader medially and laterally than centrally. Considered inharmonious and not recommended.
5. Broader centrally than medially and laterally. Considered inharmonious and not recommended.

A broad crease (>10 mm) was advocated by Song for people with a rectangular face and a strong character, such as performers and actors. An average crease (7–8 mm) is chosen most often. A narrow crease (4–5 mm) is recommended for people who want a crease but are self-conscious about others knowing about the operation. A nasally tapered crease and a parallel crease based on tarsal height give the face the most aesthetic harmony.

The conclusion is similar to what the author stated a year earlier in 1987,[22] i.e. that a nasally tapered crease and a parallel crease based on tarsal height measurement give the best aesthetic appearance to the face.[13]

Summary

It is apparent that there is more than a superficial difference between Asian and Caucasian eyelids. In addition to the readily apparent differences in the size of the lids, crease shape, and crease height, there are also anatomic differences in the tarsus and fat pads, differences in the structure of the medial canthus, differences in facial configuration, and differences in the concept of beauty. All these factors should be taken into account in the performance of Asian blepharoplasty.

References

1. Millard DR Jr. Oriental peregrinations. Plast Reconstr Surg 1955;16:319–336.
2. Millard DR Jr. The oriental eyelid and its surgical revision. Am J Ophthalmol 1964;57:646–649.
3. Chen WPD. Upper blepharoplasty in the Asian patient. In: Putterman AM, ed. Cosmetic oculoplastic surgery, 3rd edn. Philadelphia: WB Saunders, 2000: Chapter 11.
4. Chen WPD. Review of Aguilar G. Complications of oriental blepharoplasty. In: Mauriello J, ed. Management and avoidance of complications of eyelid surgery. Vol. 3. Philadelphia: Field & Wood, 1994.

5. Doxanas MT, Anderson RL. Oriental eyelids: anatomic studies. Arch Ophthalmol 1984;102:1232–1235.

6. Jeong S, Lemke B, Dortzbach R. Comparison of Asian and Caucasian upper eyelid. Arch Ophthalmol 1999;117:907–912.

7. Anderson RL, Beard C. The levator aponeurosis. Arch Ophthalmol 1977;95:1437–1441.

8. Collin JR, Beard C, Wood I. Experimental and clinical data on the insertion of the levator palpebrae superioris muscle. Am J Ophthalmol 1978;85:792–801.

9. Cheng J, Xu Feng-Zhi. Anatomic microstructure of the upper eyelid in the oriental double eyelid. Plast Reconstruct Surg 2001;107: 1665–1668.

10. Morikawa K, Yamamoto H, Uchinuma E, Yamashina S. Scanning electron microscopic study on double and single eyelids in Orientals. Aesth Plast Surg 2001;25:20–24.

11. Hwang K, Kim DJ, Chung RS, Lee SI, Hiraga Y. An anatomical study of the junction of the orbital septum and the levator aponeurosis in Orientals. Br J Plast Surg 1998;51:594–598.

12. Fink WH. An anatomic study of the check mechanism of the vertical muscles of the eyes. Am J Ophthalmol 1957;44:800–811.

13. Bang YH, Chu HH, Park SH, Kim JH, Cho JW, Kim YS. The fallacy of the levator expansion theory. Plast Reconstruct Surg 1999;103: 1788–1791.

14. Boo-Chai K. [Discussion following above paper by Bang.] Plast Reconstruct Surg 1999;103: 1792–1793.

15. Uchida J. A surgical procedure for blepharoptosis vera and for pseudo-blepharoptosis orientalis. Br J Plast Surg 1962;15:271–276.

16. Miyake I, Tange I, Hirage Y. MRI findings of the upper eyelid and their relationship with single and double-eyelid formation. Aesth Plast Surg 1994;88:183–187.

17. Yoo HB. The double eyelid operation without supratarsal fixation. Plast Reconstruct Surg 1991;88:12–17.

18. Johnson CC. Epicanthus. Am J Ophthalmol 1968;66:939–946.

19. Boo-Chai K. The Mongolian fold (plica Mongolia). Singapore Med J 1962;3:132–136.

20. Lessa S, Sebastia R. Z-epicanthoplasty. Aesth Plast Surg 1984;8:159–163.

21. del Campo AF. Surgical treatment of the epicanthal fold. Plast Reconstr Surg 1984;73:566–570.

22. Chen WPD. Asian blepharoplasty. Ophthalmol Plast Reconstr Surg 1987;3:135–140.

23. Chen WPD. A comparison of Caucasian and Asian blepharoplasty. Ophthalm Pract 191;9:216–222.

24. Kawai K, Imanishi N, Nakajima H, et al. Arterial anatomic features of the upper palpebra. Plast Reconstruct Surg 2004;113:479–484.

25. Kim BG, Youn DY, Yoon ES, et al. Unexpected bleeding caused by arterial variation inferolateral to levator palpebrae. Aesth Plast Surg 2003;27:123–125.

26. Hwang K, Kim BG, Kim YJ, Chung IH. Lateral septoaponeurotic artery: source of bleeding in blepharoplasty performed in Asians. Ann Plast Surg 2003;50:16–159.

27. Onizuka T, Iwanami M. Blepharoplasty in Japan. Aesth Plast Surg 1984;8:97–100.

28. Song RY. Further comment on double eyelid operation. [In Chinese] Chin J Plast Surg Burns 1988;4:6–9.

Upper Lid Crease – Terminology and Configurations

Chapter 3

William P.D. Chen

The configuration of the upper lid crease in Asians varies greatly. The terminology used to describe these configurations also varies, depending on the ethnic group and language concerned. Figure 3-1 illustrates the Chinese characters for the words 'double-eyelid fold'. Figure 3-2 shows the Japanese Kanji writing for 'single (one) lid eye' and 'double (two) lid eye'. The characters common to Chinese and Japanese for the operation to construct a lid crease are illustrated in Figure 3-3.

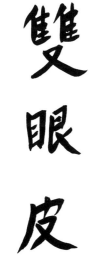

Fig. 3-1 Chinese written characters for 'double eyelid (skin)'.

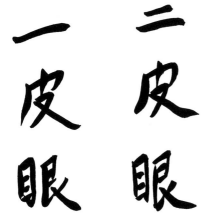

Fig. 3-2 Japanese Kanji characters for 'single eyelid,' (left) and 'double (two) eyelid' (right).

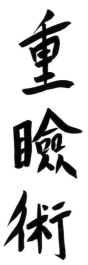

Fig. 3-3 Characters common to Chinese and Japanese for the procedure to construct an eyelid crease, or 'double-eyelid procedure'.

As described in previous publications by the author,[1–9] the crease may be asymmetric in its presentation, or be absent in one eye and present in the other. It may be continuous or segmented (fragmented).

Figure 3-4 shows the various configurations of the Asian eyelid.

Figure 3-5 shows an eyelid without a crease. There is mild degree of upper lid hooding, causing secondary downward rotation of the lashes. Figure 3-6 illustrates an eyelid with a distinctive crease. This is the parallel configuration. Figure 3-7 is an eyelid in which a portion of the crease has been obliterated. An eyelid with an incomplete or partial crease is shown in Figure 3-8. The crease originates in the medial canthus and medial upper lid fold (supracanthal web) and extends halfway across the upper lid. Multiple creases are illustrated in Figure 3-9, where two well-defined creases run parallel to each other. Figure 3-10 shows a minimal nasally tapered crease. The lateral third of the crease may be the same distance from the eyelash margin as the central third, or it may rise slightly to form

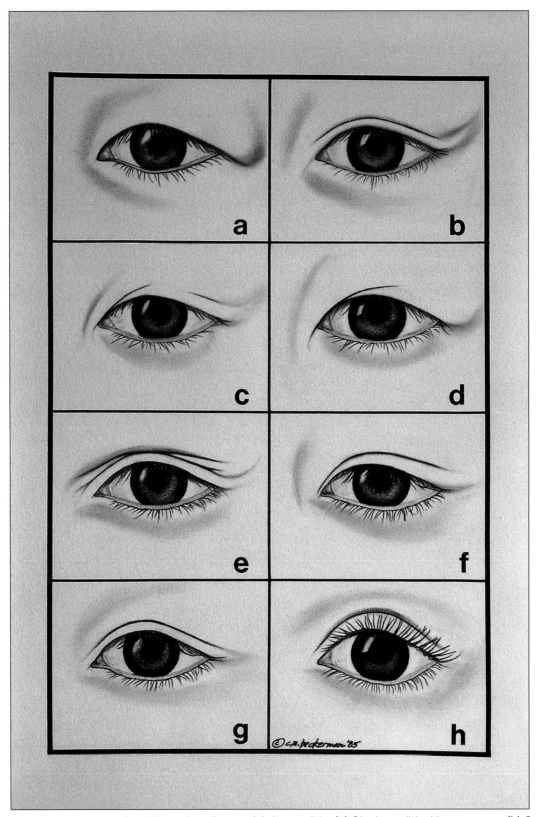

Fig. 3-4 Chen[1] has previously described the various forms of Asian eyelids: **(a)** Single eyelid without crease. **(b)** Same size eyelid fissure with crease. **(c)** Segmented or non-continuous crease. **(d)** Partial or incomplete crease. **(e)** Multiple creases. **(f)** Asian eyelid with a nasally tapered crease; in a small percentage of cases it shows some lateral flare. **(g)** Asian eyelid with a parallel crease. **(h)** Typical Caucasian semilunar crease.

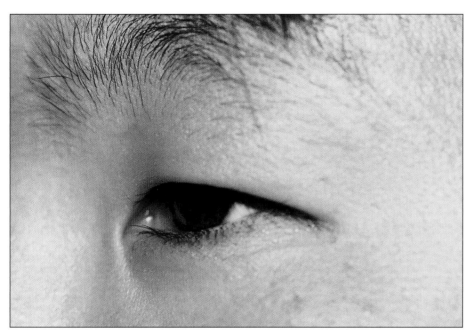

Fig. 3-5 Asian lid without crease. This patient has moderate upper lid hooding causing downward rotation of the lashes. Note the apparent upper lid hooding (fold) that overshadows the smaller palpebral fissure laterally. Strategic placement of a crease would make the palpebral fissure seem larger.

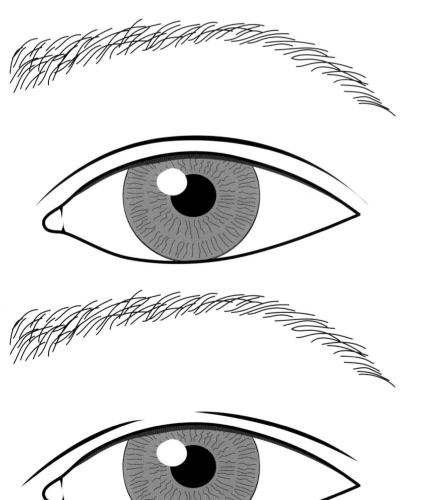

Fig. 3-6 Asian eyelid with a parallel crease.

Fig. 3-7 Partial obliteration of crease.

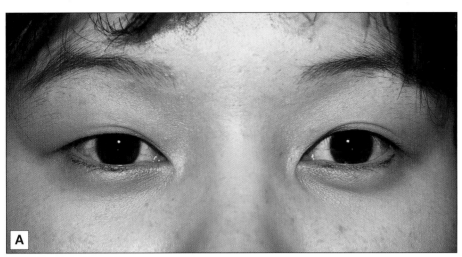

Fig. 3-8(A, B) Incomplete or partial crease.

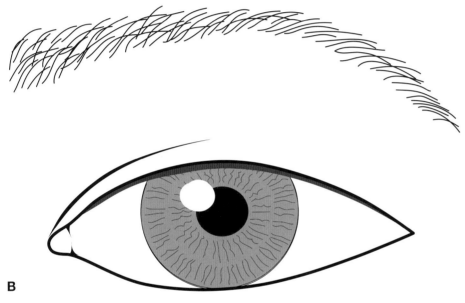

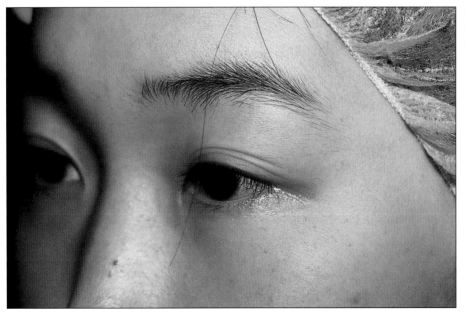

Fig. 3-9 Asian with two well-defined creases that run parallel to each other but in a nasally tapered configuration.

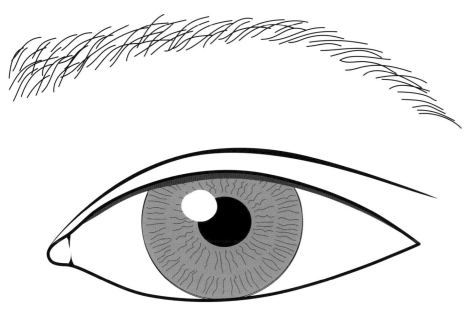

Fig. 3-10 Minimal nasally tapered crease with a mild lateral flare.

a laterally flared crease, in which the lateral third of the crease is further from the lash margin than the central third. A Caucasian upper lid crease is shown in Figure 3-11, where the central third of the crease is farthest from the lash margin.

In Asians with a continuous eyelid crease, the crease may be of the nasally tapering type (NTC) (a less desirable term is 'inside' fold) in which the crease converges toward the medial canthus, coming closer to the lashes as it reaches the medial canthal angle (Fig. 3-12A), or it may be a parallel crease (PC) (a less desirable term is 'outside' fold), in which the crease runs fairly parallel to the lash margin from the medial canthus to the lateral canthus (Fig. 3-12B).

In eyelids with a nasally tapered crease the crease may gently flare away from the lid margin as it approaches the lateral canthal region, forming a laterally flared crease (LTC) (Fig. 3-13). Another configuration is that the nasally tapering crease may run level to the eyelash margin from the central third of the eyelid laterally (Fig. 3-14).

Asians rarely have a lid crease that is semilunar in shape, as is common in Caucasians (see Figs. 3-4 and 2-5). In a semilunar crease each end of the crease is closer to the respective lid margin than the central portion of the crease. Having a semilunar crease is by far the most frequent complaint heard from Asian patients who have had blepharoplasty performed in the United States[2] (Fig. 3-15). This crease is often too high, unnatural, and harsh (termed the 'huh' syndrome).

A high crease is one located 10–12 mm from the ciliary margin. A high crease may result if a surgeon adheres to an empiric formula for the height of the lid crease, or uses techniques of supratarsal fixation in which a distance of 10 mm or more is applied without regard to ethnicity. Either method results in a crease that looks excessively high on an Asian patient. To summarize, such a regimented approach is counter-effective in Asian blepharoplasty for the following reasons:

- Asians are usually smaller in build; correspondingly, the upper tarsus measures only 6.5–8.5 mm in height on average.
- The distance between the eyebrow and the upper lid margin is smaller on Asians than on Caucasians. A crease located 10–12 mm from the lash margin would look much closer to the mid level of the upper lid than is natural (Fig. 3-16).

Not only should ethnicity be a factor in blepharoplasty, but also each individual's features. When the crease is high, it is farther from the lid margin than the height of the tarsus, the surgically applied crease traverses thick dermis as it approaches the brow and is likely to be associated with hypertrophic scarring. The large distance between the lash margin and the crease also allows little camouflage by the upper eyelashes, and the crease is exposed to scrutiny. A crease is harsh when it

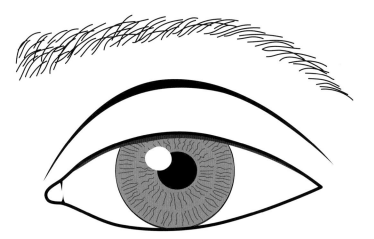

Fig. 3-11 Caucasian upper lid crease with a semilunar shape. Note that the widest separation of the crease from the ciliary border occurs centrally.

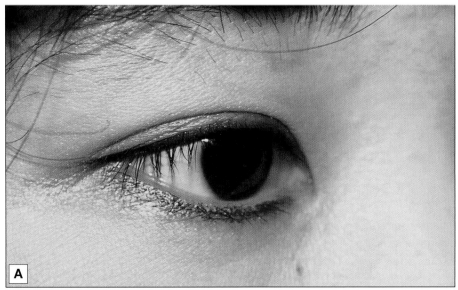

Fig. 3-12 (A) Asian eyelid with a nasally tapered crease. Note the merging of the crease medially into the medial upper lid fold and the relatively parallel course from the central third of the lid outward. **(B)** Asian eyelid with a parallel crease.

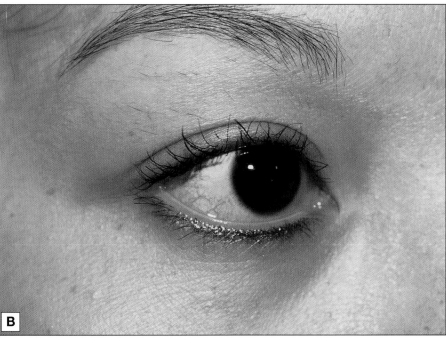

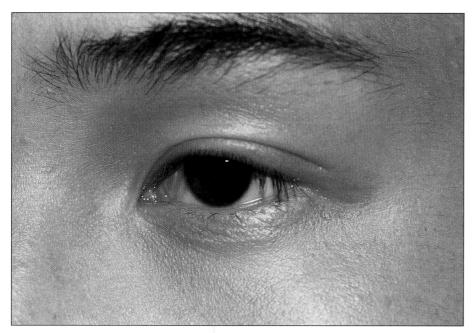

Fig. 3-13 Nasally tapered crease with a lateral flare. The widest separation of the crease from the ciliary border occurs laterally.

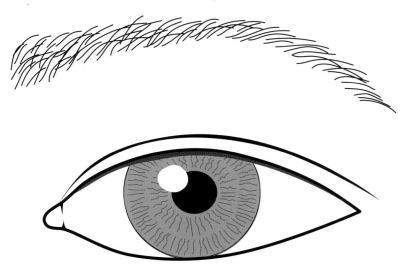

Fig. 3-14 Nasally tapered crease that runs level to the eyelash from the central third of the eyelid outward (see Fig. 3-12A).

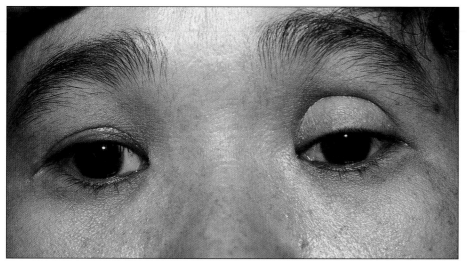

Fig. 3-15 Asian patient after blepharoplasty. Note asymmetry of the two creases and the high placement of the semilunar crease.

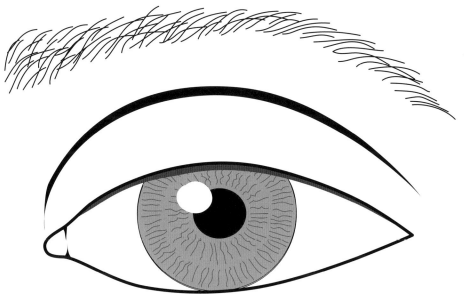

Fig. 3-16 When a semilunar crease is placed more than 10–12 mm in an Asian upper lid, the crease is in the mid level of the eyelid, halfway to the brow.

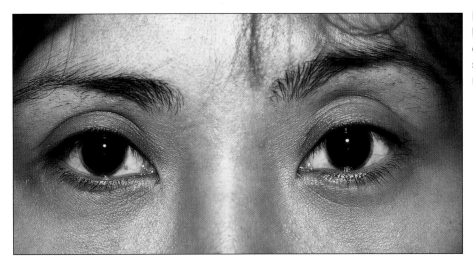

Fig. 3-17 Asian patient who underwent blepharoplasty with excessive removal of preaponeurotic fat. Note the hollow supratarsal sulcus and the formation of multiple creases.

is overtly prominent, deep, and indurated with dermal reaction.

An unnatural crease describes a shape that is not aesthetically pleasing on the face of the person. The most frequent complaint is a semilunar crease. The overall impression of a crease positioned high and semilunar in shape is unnatural for Asians. Removal of an excessive amount of preaponeurotic fat also can cause an unnatural crease. When all the fat pads are removed from the preaponeurotic space, the result is a hollowed eye or 'famined' look that appears incongruous on the relatively flat face of an Asian[2] (Fig. 3-17). For Caucasians, the same complete excision of preaponeurotic fat pads used to be a necessary step in the performance of a total cosmetic blepharoplasty.

It is important to recognize that there is a high degree of variation in the anatomy of the upper eyelids of Asians. A common misconception is that all Asians are born without an upper lid crease. In fact, half the Asian population does have a natural crease. For each person, the shape and height of the crease and the relation of the crease to facial configuration should be part of the overall assessment before a cosmetic surgical procedure is performed.

References

1. Chen WPD. Asian blepharoplasty. Ophthalmol Plast Reconstruct Surg 1987;3:135–140.
2. Chen WPD. Review of Aguilar G. Complications of oriental blepharoplasty. In: Mauriello J, ed. Management and avoidance of complications of eyelid surgery. Vol. 3. Philadelphia: Field & Wood, 1994.
3. Chen WPD. Concept of triangular, rectangular and trapezoidal debulking of eyelid tissues: application in Asian blepharoplasty. Plast Reconstruct Surg 1996;97:212–218.
4. Chen WPD. Eyelid and eyelid skin diseases. In: Lee D, Higginbotham E, eds. Clinical guide to comprehensive ophthalmology. Stuttgart: Thieme, 1999: 137–182.
5. Chen WPD. Upper eyelid blepharoplasty in the Asian patient. In: Putterman AM, ed. Cosmetic oculoplastic surgery, 3rd edn. Philadelphia: WB Saunders, 1999: 101–111.
6. Chen WPD. Expert commentary on blepharoplasty and blepharoptosis surgery in Asians. In: Mauriello J, ed. Unfavorable results of eyelid and lacrimal surgery. Oxford: Butterworth–Heinemann, 2000: 68–71.
7. Chen WPD. Aesthetic eyelid surgery in Asians: an East–West view. Hong Kong J Ophthalmol 2000;3:27–31.
8. Chen WPD. Oculoplastic surgery – the essentials. Stuttgart: Thieme, 2001.
9. Chen WPD, Khan J, McCord C. Color atlas of cosmetic oculoplastic surgery. Oxford: Butterworth–Heinemann, 2004.

Preoperative Counseling

Chapter 4

William P.D. Chen

Most patients who request Asian blepharoplasty are Chinese, Japanese, Korean, Filipino or Southeast Asian. It is important to note that in these ethnic groups more than half of the overall population has an upper lid crease. A patient seeking a consultation is likely not to have a lid crease, and it is important to be aware that they want a crease so that they may look like their fellow Asians, not Caucasian.

It is crucial to be aware that there may be errors in communication and misunderstanding between surgeon and patient.[1] This is especially critical at the first meeting, when the surgeon tries to determine the patient's needs and to assess whether or not they can be met.

It is common and acceptable for young Japanese, Koreans, and Chinese in developed countries to undergo cosmetic eyelid operations. It is often socially acceptable for mothers to encourage their daughters to undergo the procedure, the operation not having the stigma associated with rhinoplasty, breast augmentation, or chin augmentation. Unlike these cosmetic operations, in which synthetic materials are implanted into the body (rendering the body 'not whole'), eyelid operations are perceived to be a way to improve on the beauty of the person, to 'open up' the face while being relatively non-invasive.

This attitude on the part of the patient or family is problematic when the surgeon and the patient are not communicating on the same level. Many patients who come to the author for possible correction have had the operation performed by a reputable and capable surgeon but are dissatisfied with the results. These patients complain that despite their insistence on a 'low, natural crease', the doctor gave them a high crease (Fig. 4-1); that the creases are asymmetric (Fig. 4-2); that the crease disappeared with time (Fig. 4-3); or that the surgeon gave them a hollow over the upper lid crease (usually owing to overexcision of the preaponeurotic fat pads) (Fig. 4-4). All these unsatisfactory outcomes could be the result of the physician having his or her own perception of the operation, as in a traditional blepharoplasty, and applying it to the patient.

Patients who have suboptimal results often state afterward that they 'did not think it would be so noticeable'. Not infrequently, they may want the whole process reversed. A properly placed crease over the upper lid is natural and blends with the configuration of that particular patient's eyes and face. A suboptimal result may be very noticeable because the eyes are a focus of attention in human interaction.

Patients in the US are often bicultural and may have a preconceived perception of how the procedure might be performed. This is often their first operation of any kind. I find that most patients prefer their friends not to know they are undergoing blepharoplasty, although a large number are jubilant and tell everyone once their wounds have healed to a desirable level.

There are some prevailing patient misconceptions. Some patients expect minimal or no swelling after the operation. Some expect no sutures. Some expect no incision. Some patients expect all swelling to subside within a week. Almost all are invariably surprised at the height of the crease during the first few weeks.

As has been made apparent, crease configuration[2] is of the utmost importance to Asian patients. Crease configuration has four contributing parameters: height, shape, continuity, and permanence (Fig. 4-5).

Height

The normal height of the upper tarsus in Asians is only 6.5–8.5 mm. The clinical significance of this is that a crease positioned arbitrarily 10 mm from the ciliary margin, as suggested in some plastic surgery literature, is high for Asians.[3] Crease placement should therefore be predicated on measuring the true anatomic height of the upper tarsus on the patient in question; this should be used as a relative guideline in defining where the crease should be positioned.

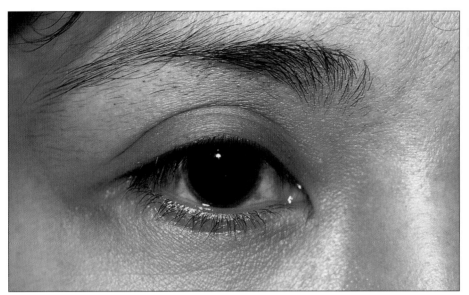

Fig. 4-1 Results after blepharoplasty show multiple high, semilunar creases caused by excessive removal of preaponeurotic fat.

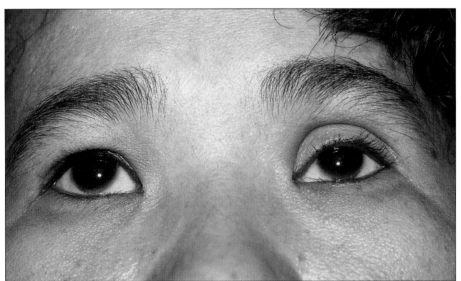

Fig. 4-2 Postoperative asymmetric crease.

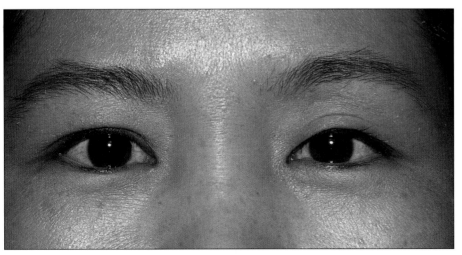

Fig. 4-3 Fading of surgically constructed crease in the left upper lid.

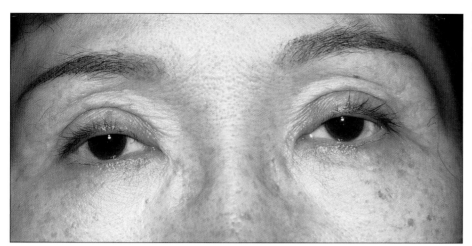

Fig. 4-4 Elderly patient after blepharoplasty in which excessive fat was removed. Note the presence of multiple creases and folds.

Fig. 4-5 Interrelated parameters of the configuration of an eyelid crease.

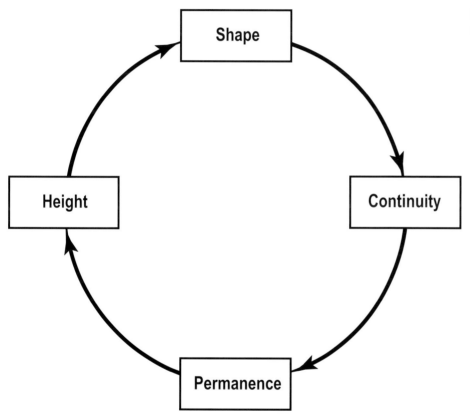

The author informs the patient that a properly applied crease will invariably appear high postoperatively because of tissue swelling (Fig. 4-6). Patients are told to expect postoperative edema to last for at least 10 days, and that the crease configuration may vary from month to month and from one eyelid to the other. Patients are instructed not to expect a stable and satisfactory appearance until 2 months after the operation. I find that preparing patients adequately makes them a lot more accepting of the normal wound healing process.

Shape

The shape of the crease must be discussed with the patient before the operation. A large percentage of patients know what they want in terms of crease configuration and its degree of prominence. Patients who do not know are informed of the desirability of a nasally tapered or parallel crease and the undesirability of a semilunar crease, which is truly an occidental crease and appears incongruous on an Asian face. The ultimate decision, of course, rests with the patient.

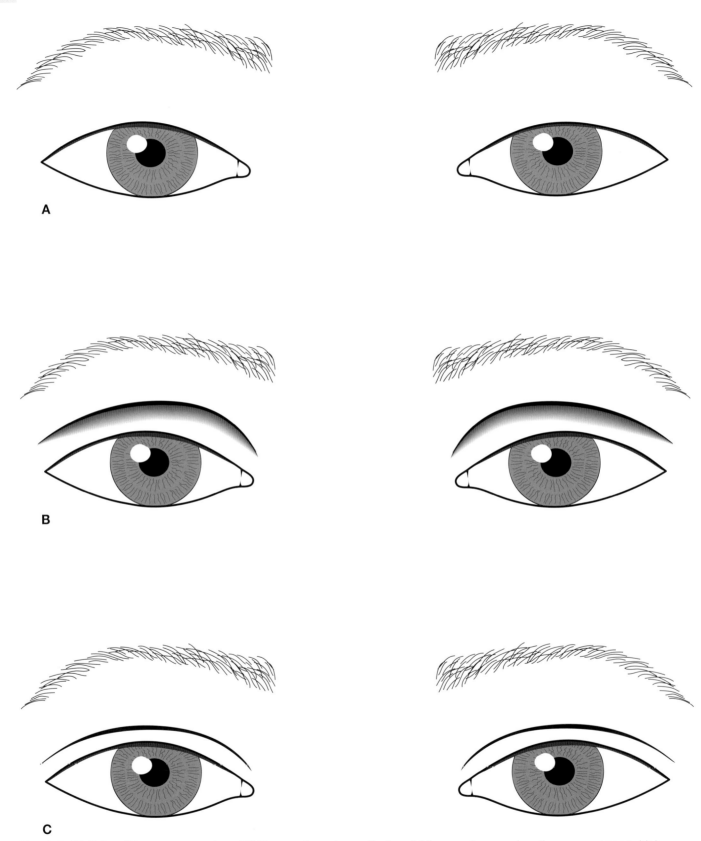

Fig. 4-6 (A) Before lid crease procedure. **(B)** One week postoperatively, mild tissue edema makes the crease appear high. **(C)** Two months postoperatively. The resolution of pretarsal fullness cause apparent downward migration of the crease.

None of the author's patients has chosen a semilunar crease after the different configurations and their prevalence in Asians have been explained.

Of the two parameters above, I would say that height is actually more important for the surgeon to be critically accurate, whereas patients are typically concerned with the shape of the desired crease.

Continuity and Permanence

Continuity and permanence are surgical goals that the author tries to achieve in all operations. After the operation, the crease should be continuous along the width of the eyelid fissure without any interruption or multiplicity. To be considered permanent, the crease should be present well beyond 24 months after the operation: even though a great number of techniques are discussed in the literature, not all of them have predictable and long-lasting results.

In my first office consultation with a new patient, I listen first to their complaints and mentally classify them into a relative order (or wish-list) of those that can be improved upon as opposed to a transient improvement or no improvement at all. Ultimately both the surgeon and the patient need to agree on what is comfortable, beneficial and worthwhile for the patient. I always try to encourage patients to speak their mind, even if they may be embarrassed, and to facilitate this in a stress-free environment. Very often patients may be overly self-conscious about an issue that matters little to anyone they interact with, or one may need to point out an extreme condition that needs to be corrected before the desired aesthetic outcome can be achieved, for example ptosis. It is important for the surgeon to customize individual aspects of their particular technique for a particular patient. I do not believe I have performed two exactly identical procedures in any of my Asian blepharoplasty patients.

I inform my patients that there is a 3–5% probability that they will need touch-up revisions if the creases are uneven. This is a realistic estimate in my practice, and most patients say they are comfortable with it. Other clinicians may prefer to inform their patients of a probability of touch-up revisions of 10–20%.

A basic eye examination and visual acuity is recorded for each patient. A history of dry eye symptoms is noted and highlighted. In summary, the following tasks are accomplished in the preoperative meeting with the patient:

1. The definition of and the patient's concept of a crease are discussed.
2. Crease configuration and placement are discussed.
3. The surgical techniques to be used, including local anesthetics, sutures, and medications, are described.
4. Postoperative swelling and wound healing are explained.
5. Reasonable expectations and revisions and any possible complications are explained.
6. Signed informed consent is obtained.
7. Preoperative photographs are taken for the patient's record.
8. Preoperative instructions: avoidance of anticoagulants and herbal medications.
9. Postoperative dietary advice: do's and don'ts.
10. Postoperative eye movement exercises: timing and schedules.

The complications of Asian blepharoplasty are those that occur after any blepharoplasty. They may include hemorrhage, grossly asymmetric creases, obliteration or fading of the crease, prolonged postoperative edema, hypertrophic scar formation, and the formation of multiple creases. These complications are discussed in later chapters.

After adequate prioritization of goals with the patient, I then explain what the procedure involves before, during and after the surgery, and what is expected of the patient. This includes the mandatory preoperative cessation of aspirin products, any herbal formulas, ginseng compounds, or herbal teas, which frequently contain therapeutics with anticoagulant properties.

The patient is given a detailed written list of pre- as well as postoperative instructions, including bed rest during the first day, use of ice compresses as well as antibiotic ointments, what to expect, and instructions to call me should there be any concern.

In the patient's chart I record particular aspects of their facial structure (ptosis, brow overaction, prominent sulcus), what was mentioned to them (for example, one upper lid margin is 0.5 mm lower than the other, or one eye shows a more prominent sulcus), what was the patient's response and preferences (high crease, low crease, shape of crease line selected, as well as skin texture observed), and whether I told the patient that despite their stated preference, it might not be achievable. If a patient has thick dry skin, an oily complexion, superficial furuncles or rosacea, these are all noted on my plan of management.

Postoperative dietary recommendations are also offered to facilitate uneventful and non-inflammatory healing of the wound after the surgery (this is an aspect of traditional Chinese medicine that baffles and perplexes western medical practitioners).

In California, informed consent for surgery is mandatory and we implement it in the office as well as the outpatient surgical facilities. Patients having revision surgery sign an additional consent form detailing their understanding of the unpredictability of outcome. All patients having aesthetic surgery (for that matter, all patients in my office) must have adequate photographic documentation of their current conditions. This typically includes a frontal view, oblique side views, upgaze and downgaze and, most importantly, if the patient has had previous surgeries, a close-up macro view of the existing surgical lines or lid-crease scar. This last item has been very useful for fully informing patients in much of the revision cases I perform. In this very litigious climate, adequate documentation is truly the best policy. In the office setting I use a Sony Mavica camera, which take images in the basic 800×600 pixel range and stores them on 3.5-in floppy disks. This is conveniently kept in each patient's chart and can be used for review purposes. I use two other higher-resolution cameras for more detailed images on selective conditions when I need them for publication or teaching purposes. Currently I use a Sony Cybershot W-7 with 7 megapixels and a Nikon D-100 SLR with 5 megapixel capabilities.

If a patient seems extremely nervous I may try to call them the night before the procedure to make sure all is well. On the day of surgery, in the preoperative area, I greet the patient again and reiterate the goal(s) of the surgery. If there is any discrepancy between what I told them and what they think and expect, I would always defer the surgery until another day, although this is extremely rare.

The office staff are trained to make a follow-up telephone call to the patient the day after surgery, both to verify that the patient is stable and to confirm a return date for suture removal.

The following are a sample of preoperative advice given to patients on postoperative expectations:

1. The wound is to be cared for by local ice compression during the first 24 hours. One can expect a mild degree of swelling to start after the first day, with minimal to mild swelling over the preseptal area.
2. The swelling will start to decrease by day 4. By day 7 a normal-looking crease form will be seen at a level 40–50% higher than the eventual outcome (in other words, a perpendicularly viewed and measured crease will look like 140% of what was originally designed).
3. The swelling will have subsided by 80% by the end of 2 weeks.
4. The remaining 20% swelling will take another 6 weeks to resolve (the 80:20/2 weeks:8 weeks rule).
5. The crease height does not move: it is merely inflated up and down as wound swelling occurs and then subsides.
6. The incisional wound tension peaks at 5–6 weeks.
7. The healing wound may be pruritic. This may intensify and become reddened if the patient eats spicy and/or fried foods. Comedogenic foods such as chocolate and high-cholesterol foods such as crustaceans should be avoided as a general rule.
8. Wound induration may occur between 4 and 12 weeks postoperatively. Topical corticosteroid ointment may be prescribed as needed.
9. Minimal clinically insignificant residual swelling may linger for 6 months before total resolution.

References

1. Chen WPD. Insights from a series of Asian blepharoplasty. Presented at the 21st Annual Scientific Symposium of the American Society of Ophthalmic Plastic and Reconstructive Surgery, Atlanta, Georgia, 1990.
2. Chen WPD. Asian blepharoplasty. Ophthalmol Plast Reconstruct Surg 1987;3:135–140.
3. Chen WPD. A comparison of Caucasian and Asian blepharoplasty. Ophthalm Pract 1991;9:216–222.

Suture Ligation Methods

Chapter 5

William P.D. Chen

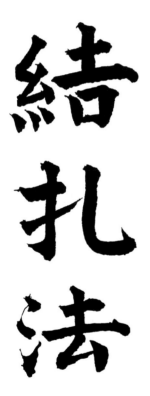

As mentioned in Chapter 1 (Historical considerations), there are two approaches to the creation of a lid crease, the suture ligation method and the external incision method. The early Japanese literature favoring the suture ligation method was discussed in that chapter and is briefly reintroduced here.

The first description of the suture ligation method, by Mikamo,[1] was published in 1896. He performed the procedure on a Japanese woman who did not have a crease in one of her upper eyelids. The crease was designed to be 6–8 mm from the ciliary margin. Three 4/0 braided silk sutures were used; these passed through the full thickness of the lid from the conjunctiva to the outer layer of skin. The depth of the crease was adjusted by the number of days the sutures were left in, the range being 2–6 days.

Uchida[2] described his suture ligation method for the double-eyelid operation. In 1926 he performed the procedure on 1523 eyelids in 396 male and 444 female patients. Uchida described the crease configuration as a fan shape, that is, a somewhat rounded crease. The crease was designed to be 7–8 mm from the ciliary margin. Three buried catgut sutures were used on each lid, encompassing approximately 2 mm of eyelid tissue horizontally. The sutures were removed 4 days after placement.

An external incision method was first mentioned in 1929, when Maruo[3] reported on both his suturing and his incision techniques. Maruo's technique required an incision across the lid, designed to be 7 mm from the ciliary margin. The wound closure technique was a trans-lid passage from the conjunctival side just above the superior tarsal border to the anterior skin surface. One 5/0 catgut suture was used to imbricate four throws along the superior tarsal border, attaching the skin edges to the underlying tarsal plate. The space between each throw was about 5–6 mm. Maruo also discussed subcutaneous dissection 5 mm superior and inferior to the incision line (see Appendix 1 for other Japanese incisional techniques from 1930 to the 1950s).

In 1954, Sayoc[4–10] first published the external incision technique in the English literature. Millard,[11] in 1955, described his Korean Armed Service experience. He mentioned that Koreans at that time desired to look 'round-eyed' like westerners, rather than 'slant eyed'. Millard believed that the absence of a crease in Koreans was a product of excess skin and supraorbital fat. One patient Millard described underwent excision of a 3-mm strip of skin, dissection under both upper and lower skin edges, trimming of the orbicularis muscles along the inferior skin incision, and complete excision of the supraorbital (preaponeurotic) fat pads. Although he used crease-enhancing silk sutures from skin to tarsus to skin, Millard believed such sutures were not always necessary. A small Z-plasty was performed selectively to eliminate an epicanthal fold. Millard's article is an interesting illustration of the interaction between western surgeons and Asian patients in the 1950s.

In 1961, Pang[12] described trans-lid placement of full-thickness eyelid sutures to form an upper lid fold. Three double-armed 4/0 silk sutures were placed from the conjunctival side toward the skin side, tied, and left in for 10 days.

Fernandez,[13] Uchida,[14] and Boo-Chai[15] also wrote articles on external incision techniques in the early 1960s. In 1962, Uchida[14] described the presence of different fat compartments and variations of fat distribution in the upper eyelids of Asians. His incision method involved the selective excision of pretarsal subcutaneous tissues, including skin, pretarsal orbicularis muscle and fat, preaponeurotic fat, and even some preseptal fat pads.

In the English literature, in 1964 Boo-Chai[15–19] advocated the simpler transconjunctival suturing technique for younger patients with minimal amounts of excess fat and skin. This was not unlike Mikamo's original method. It was followed in 1972 by Mutou and Mutou,[20] who further described the suture ligation technique (see Appendix 2: post-1950 Asian blepharoplasty). In this classic paper, the authors detailed their interpretation of their concept of the double eyelid and their less invasive method for patients with thin eyelid skin and scarce subcutaneous fat. They per-

formed 4805 cases between 1965 and 1969, of which about 10% were men. One-quarter preferred the parallel shape and three-quarters preferred the 'unfolded fan type' (equivalent to a nasally tapered crease but with gradual widening towards the lateral end of the lid fissure). To make the crease nasally tapered the authors turned the ligature over the inner canthus downward. They explained that there were three options in crease height: the lowest level at 4–5mm was called the 'deep double eyes' (the deep here connotes more of the sense of inferior anatomic location), the usual was 6–8mm, and the highest was 9–12mm and is intended for those with large eyes. The technique basically involved passing two double-armed 6/0 sutures from the conjunctival side, each traversing horizontally for 5mm at a level 3mm above the superior tarsal border in a subconjunctival fashion. Each arm is then reinserted through the conjunctiva (within 1mm of its exit) towards the skin side. One arm of the suture thus exiting on the skin side is then passed subcutaneously and tied with the second arm on the skin side. Their placement of the double-armed sutures was such that the medial ligature straddled the junction of the medial and central thirds of the upper lid; the lateral ligature straddled the lateral third of the lid. The sutures were meant to be buried permanently. The authors stated that mild transient ptosis was seen in almost all cases. They had a crease disappearance rate of 1.3% among their patients who underwent an intradermal double-eyelid procedure with buried sutures. In 1973 Mutou modified this to using a single stitch instead of two.

The suture ligation method has the advantage of being relatively non-invasive and usually causes little postoperative swelling. The main disadvantage is that the crease may disappear with time (Fig. 5-1).

In 1979, Shirakabe[21] modified Hata's 1933[22] method; Shirakabe's method consists of making an external skin incision, undermining the pretarsal area, followed by closure and crease fixation using six double-armed 4/0 nylon sutures, with each arm of each pair of the stitches looped and tied down with a small bead (total number of beads used = 12).

In a paper in 2000, Homma and Mutou[23] reported a crease regression rate of 3.4% in 1457 patients during a 7-year period from 1986. They mentioned that the technique is applicable for patients with little fat

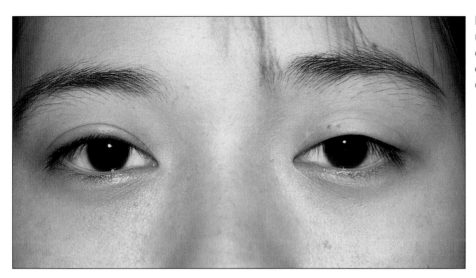

Fig. 5-1 Young Asian adult who underwent crease placement by the conjunctival suturing technique. The crease on the right is well-formed; that on the left has disappeared.

tissue or mild puffiness only. They quoted the advantages as including minimal postoperative swelling, the crease can be reversed by cutting the stitch, and no apparent scarring. The procedure involved everting the tarsus and applying a 7/0 nylon suture through the conjunctiva at a point 3 mm above the superior tarsal border, traversing the conjunctiva for 5 mm. One arm is reinserted through the conjunctiva 1 mm adjacent to where it came out, exiting through the anterior skin surface. This is followed by the second arm of the conjunctival suture, exiting the skin in the same fashion. The first suture is then passed subcutaneously to join the second suture, now on the skin side, and the two are tied and cut close to the knot.

Other authors, including Tsurukiri,[24] reported a regression rate of 10%. Satou and Ichida[25] reported a regression rate of 16.8%. Homma and Mutou[23] postulated that the disappearance rate is higher in individuals with thicker skin or who possess excess subcutaneous fat. They acknowledged the difficulty of assessing the true rate of disappearance, as patients often do not return for follow-up and often seek other doctors for revision when the first procedure is suboptimal. A significant factor not discussed is the fact that most patients who undergo the stitch methods realize that when the crease does disappear they are often candidates for the incision method, and therefore may proceed to seek consultation directly with those who practice the open incision method.

There are other papers describing the use of small incisional approach with the removal of tissues along the superior tarsal area, together with the passage of buried sutures. For example, Lee et al.[26] described the use of 7/0 nylon through small skin incisions, applying it as a buried figure-of-eight continuous suture forming three hexagonal loops spanning the width of the crease; this was combined with removal of tissue (muscle, preseptal fat, and septum). They used this technique in 327 patients with a mean follow-up of 13 months only.

From 1970 to 1990 at least a dozen articles describing the external incision methods were published (see Appendix 2). Zubiri's[27] article in 1981 described measurement of the vertical dimension of the upper tarsus as a way to guide placement of the lid crease incision. I favor this method because it is a logical and anatomically correct way to tailor the incision lines and because it approximates the true position of the crease.

The wealth of information from earlier clinical practitioners helped lay the foundation for the continued evolution of cosmetic upper eyelid surgery for Asians. During the 12 years since the first edition of this book was published there have been at least an additional 22 publications, whose topics included epicanthoplasty as well as papers describing smaller skin incisions or 'partial' incision variations of the external incision techniques, and various forms of crease fixation, including 'septodermal' and 'orbicularis–levator' fixation.

The rest of this chapter will now concentrate on the suture ligation method. Almost all the published papers on suture ligation methods can be subcategorized into six variations.

Suture Ligation Method

In this technique the goal is to create adhesions between the levator aponeurosis along the superior tarsal border and the subdermal tissue overlying it without making a significant skin incision.

The eyelid is first anesthetized by local infiltration of lidocaine hydrochloride. The upper eyelid is everted, and three double-armed sutures are placed from the conjunctival side (transconjunctival) in a subconjunctival fashion above the superior tarsal border (Step 1). One of the following three alternative steps may be performed to complete this procedure.

Variation 1: Full-Thickness Suture Technique

Both ends of the suture pass through to the skin surface (Step 2); one end is then passed subcutaneously again to exit through the exit site of the second needle on the skin (Step 3). The two ends are tied and buried subcutaneously (Fig. 5-2).

Variation 2: Full-Thickness Suture Technique with Stab Skin Incisions

One end of the suture passes through the lid and exits through a stab skin incision (Step 2). The other end goes through skin next to the stab incision and is repassed subcutaneously to join the first suture, which exited through the stab incision (Step 3). The two ends of the suture are tied in the stab incision and buried (see Boo-Chai[17] and Appendix 2). As in Alternative 1, the suture knot encompasses the Müller muscle, levator aponeurosis, and some pretarsal orbicularis oculi muscle, producing a scar or a tightening process between the subdermal tissues along the superior tarsal border and the levator aponeurosis–Müller muscle complex (Fig. 5-3).

Variation 3: Transconjunctival Intramuscular Suture Technique

Without piercing the skin, one end of the double-armed suture is passed through the Müller muscle and levator aponeurosis to the subcutaneous plane along the superior tarsal border. The needle remains in the subcutaneous plane; the suture arm is reversed through the same tissue and exits through the conjunctiva (Step 2). The two ends of the suture are knotted and buried within the conjunctiva above the superior tarsal border. Some surgeons prefer to cut out a small piece of tarsus and bury the knot within the space to prevent corneal or conjunctival irritation (Fig. 5-4).

There are three other variations of the suture ligation method worthy of discussion. Approaching from the skin side, they are discussed below.

Variation 4: Transcutaneous Intramuscular Suture Technique (Without Piercing the Conjunctiva)

Two small stab incisions are made on the skin side at the level of the eyelid crease. Sutures of 6/0 nylon or polypropylene are passed from the first stab incision through levator aponeurosis and some Müller muscle. The suture material is then passed a short distance along the proposed level of the crease before being returned on the skin side through the second stab incision (Step 1). The other end of the suture is repassed subcutaneously to join the first half of the suture in the second stab incision; it is then tied and buried subcutaneously (Step 2) (Fig. 5-5). Mutou and Mutou[20] used two of these sutures to form the crease (see Appendix 2).

Variation 5: Twisted Needle and Compression Method (Transcutaneous and Intratarsal Suturing with Twisted Needle Tracking Method)

In China, Yang[27] made several stab incisions along the superior tarsal border (Fig. 5-6A). A needle with screw threads (or an equivalent tool, such as a no. 6 root canal dental file; Fig. 5-6D) is twirled through the subcutaneous plane and then through the suborbicularis plane along the pretarsal region of the upper lid (step A in illustration), first from the lateral to the central stab incision and then from the central to the medial incision. Sutures of 4/0 silk are then used to close the wound in a continuous manner, taking a bite of the tarsus and passing back to the skin side, as in steps B or

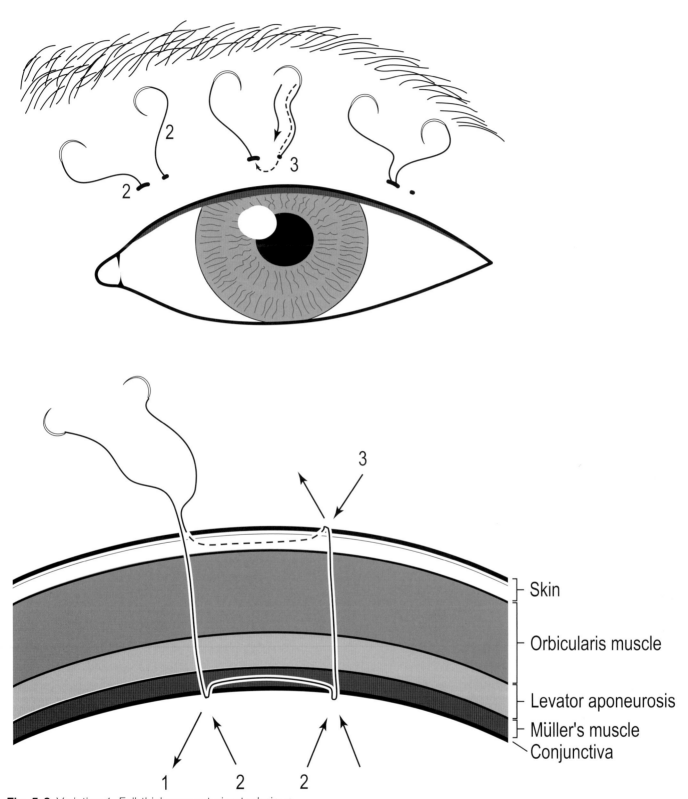

Fig. 5-2 Variation 1. Full-thickness suturing technique.

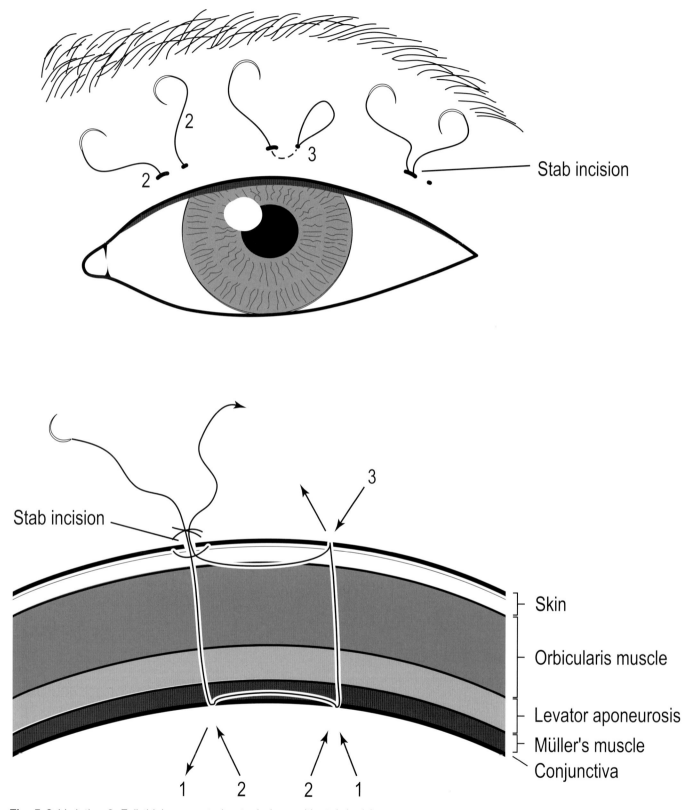

Fig. 5-3 Variation 2. Full-thickness suturing technique with stab incisions.

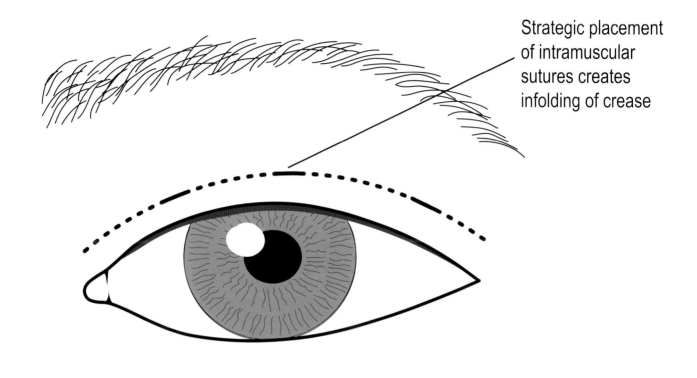

Strategic placement of intramuscular sutures creates infolding of crease

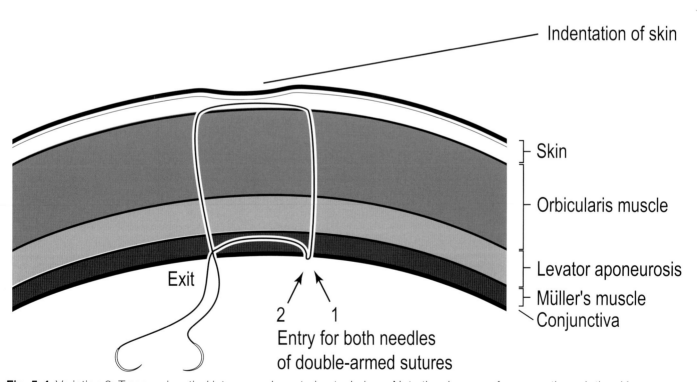

Indentation of skin

Skin

Orbicularis muscle

Levator aponeurosis

Müller's muscle

Conjunctiva

Exit

2   1

Entry for both needles of double-armed sutures

Fig. 5-4 Variation 3. Transconjunctival intramuscular suturing technique. Note the absence of passage through the skin.

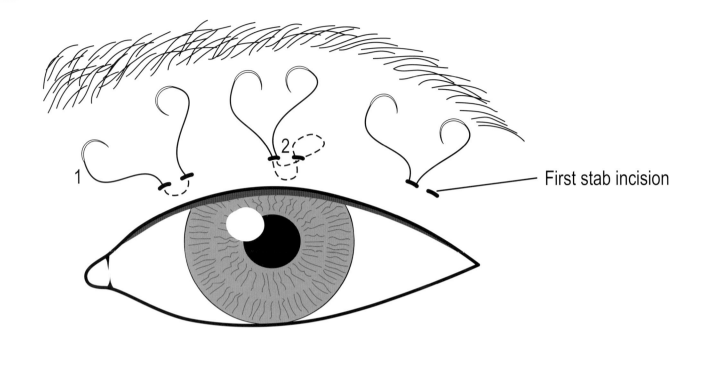

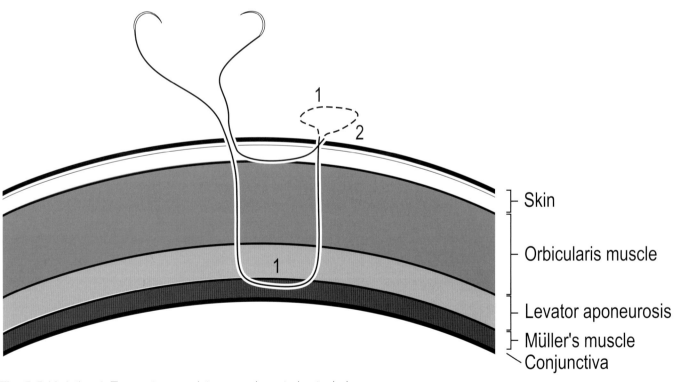

Fig. 5-5 Variation 4. Transcutaneous intramuscular suturing technique.

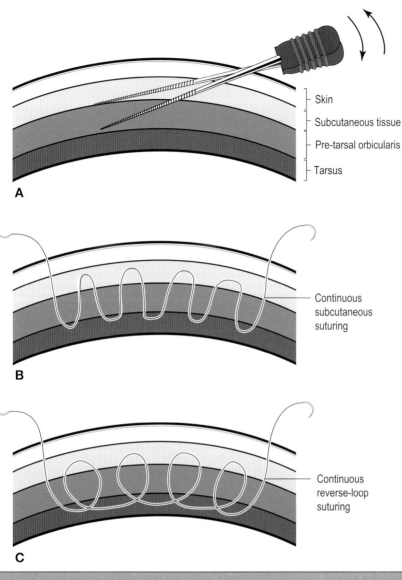

Skin

Subcutaneous tissue

Pre-tarsal orbicularis

Tarsus

A

Continuous
subcutaneous
suturing

B

Continuous
reverse-loop
suturing

C

Fig. 5-6 Variation 5. (Top) Twisted needle and compression technique with transcutaneous intratarsal suturing. (Bottom) Root canal dental files.

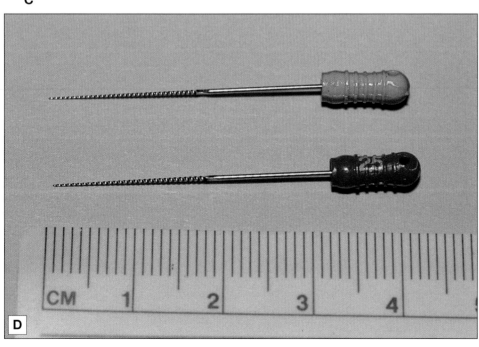

D

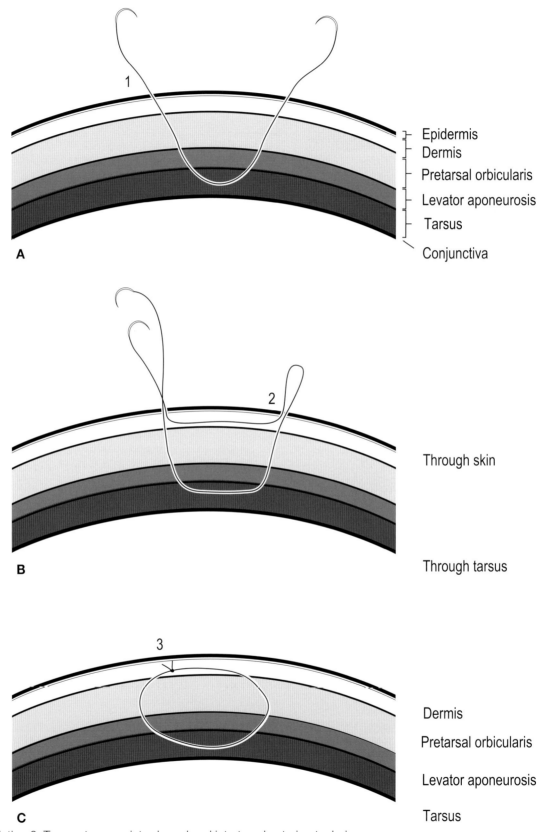

Fig. 5-7 Variation 6. Transcutaneous intradermal and intratarsal suturing technique.

C. At the same time, a half-section of a rubber catheter about 2 mm wide is sutured across the pretarsal region. It is postulated that scarring caused by passage of the screw-threaded needle and the compressive effect of the rubber catheter causes aponeurosis–subcutaneous attachment and formation of the lid crease.

Yang reported that the advantages of this procedure include rapid resolution of postoperative edema and swelling and the lack of an open skin incision. Yang reported the procedure to be effective for 100 of 102 patients 3 years postoperatively. Contraindications to the procedure include excessive fat, scarcity of skin, or an excess of dermatochalasis. The technique is not suitable for patients with lid retraction or prominent palpebral fissures, or those undergoing reoperation.

Variation 6: Transcutaneous Intradermal and Intratarsal Suturing Technique

In China, Song[28] reported a variation in which a no. 11 blade is used to make two stab incisions 3–5 mm apart over the medial, central, and lateral thirds of the upper lid; the incisions extend down to the tarsal plate from the skin (Fig. 5-7). One end of a suture needle is passed from one stab incision on the skin through the tarsal plate superficially and exits through the second stab incision (Step 1). The second needle enters through the same stab incision used by the first, this time tracking intradermally and exiting through the second stab wound, as did the first needle (Step 2). The sutures are tied and buried in the subcutaneous plane (Step 3). The previous steps are repeated over each third of the superior tarsal border. According to Song, it is important to make sure that the sutures track intradermally rather than subcutaneously, because when subcutaneous sutures are used the crease tends to disappear soon after the operation.

In alternatives 3, 4, and 6, both needles enter and exit through the same points on the eyelid. Alternatives 4, 5, and 6 involve transcutaneous passage. Alternatives 5 and 6 involve intratarsal passage.

Even though these suture ligation techniques avoid making wide skin incisions, four of the six options (with the exception of alternatives 1 and 3) require several stab incisions through the skin or multiple needle passages through the skin surface.

References

1. Mikamo K. A technique in the double eyelid operation. J Chugaishinpo 1896.
2. Uchida K. The Uchida method for the double-eyelid operation in 1523 cases. Jpn J Ophthalmol 1926;30:593.
3. Maruo M. Plastic construction of a 'double-eyelid'. Jpn Rev Clin Ophthalmol 1929;24:393–406.
4. Sayoc BT. Plastic construction of the superior palpebral fold. Am J Ophthalmol 1954;38:556–559.
5. Sayoc BT. Simultaneous construction of the superior palpebral fold in ptosis operation. Am J Ophthalmol 1956;41:1040–1043.
6. Sayoc BT. Absence of superior palpebral fold in slit eyes (an anatomic and physiologic explanation). Am J Ophthalmol 1956;42:298–300.
7. Sayoc BT. Surgical management of unilateral almond eye. Am J Ophthalmol 1961;52:122.
8. Sayoc BT. Blepharo-dermachalasis. Am J Ophthalmol 1962;53:1020–1022.
9. Sayoc BT. Anatomic considerations in the plastic construction of a palpebral fold in the full upper eyelid. Am J Ophthalmol 1967;63:155–158.
10. Sayoc BT. Surgery of the oriental eyelid. Clin Plast Surg 1974;1:157–171.
11. Millard DR Jr. Oriental peregrinations. Plast Reconstruct Surg 1955;16:319–336.
12. Pang HG. Surgical formation of upper lid fold. Arch Ophthalmol 1961;65:783–784.
13. Fernandez LR. Double eyelid operation in the Oriental in Hawaii. Plast Reconstruct Surg 1960;25:257–264.
14. Uchida J. A surgical procedure for blepharoptosis vera and for pseudo-blepharoptosis orientalis. Br J Plast Surg 1962;15:271–276.
15. Boo-Chai K. Plastic construction of the superior palpebral fold. Plast Reconstruct Surg 1963;31:74–78.
16. Boo-Chai K. Further experience with cosmetic surgery of the upper eyelid. In: Broadbent TR, ed. Transactions of the Third International Congress of Plastic Surgery. Amsterdam: Excerpta Medica, 1964: 518–524.

17. Boo-Chai K. Some aspects of plastic (cosmetic) surgery in Orientals. Br J Plast Surg 1969;22:60–69.

18. Boo-Chai K. Aesthetic surgery for the Oriental. In:Barron JN, Saad MN, eds. Operative plastic and reconstructive surgery. Vol. 2. Edinburgh: Churchill Livingstone, 1980: 761–781.

19. Boo-Chai K. Surgery for the oriental eyelid. In: Lewis JR Jr, ed. The art of aesthetic plastic surgery. Boston: Little, Brown, 1989: 611–617.

20. Mutou Y, Mutou H. Intradermal double eyelid operation and its follow-up results. Br J Plast Surg 1972;25:285–291.

21. Shirakabe Y. Mikamo's double-eyelid operation: The advent of Japanese aesthetic surgery. Plast Reconstr Surg 1997;99:668–669.

22. Hata B. Application of eyelid clamp and beads in 'double-eyelid' operation. Jpn Rev Clin Ophthalmol 1933;28:491–494.

23. Homma K, Mutou Y, Mutou H, Ezoe K, Fujita T. Intradermal stitch for orientals: does it disappear? Aesth Plast Surg 2000;24:289–291.

24. Tsurukiri K. Double eyelid plasty: reliability and unfavorable results to the patients [Abstract]. J Jpn Aesth Plast Surg 1999;20:38.

25. Satou H, Ichida M. The reliability of buried double eyelid operation and the assessment of unfavorable results at our clinic. Panel discussion at the annual meeting of the Japan Society of Aesthetic Plastic Surgery, Gifu, Japan, October 1998.

26. Lee YJ, Baek RM, Chung WJ. Nonincisional blepharoplasty using the debulking method. Aesth Plast Surg 2004;27:434–437.

27. Zubiri JS. Correction of the oriental eyelid. Clin Plast Surg 1981;8:725–737.

28. Yang PY. Double eyelid operation by the twisted needle and compressive suturing technique. Clin J Plast Surg Burns 1987;3:191–192.

29. Song RY. Further discussion on the improved suturing technique for double eyelid operation (intradermal and intratarsal suturing technique). Chin J Plast Surg Burn 1990;6:96–97.

External Incision Methods

William P.D. Chen

Chapter 6

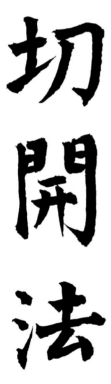

A review of the literature on the external incision method (see Appendix 2) shows considerable variations in technique and preference regarding skin incisions and whether or not skin and orbicularis muscle should be routinely removed. Likewise, some prefer to open the orbital septum and remove a variable amount of the preaponeurotic fat pad.

There are other proponents for small skin incisions or partial incision only, and further differentiations in the way crease fixation is carried out, including skin–levator aponeurosis–skin, inferior orbicularis–levator, septodermal, and skin–tarsus–skin fixation. Each variation has pros and cons that needs to be weighed according to the technical skills, aesthetic sense and level of effort involved, as well as the patient's comfort level and acceptance.

For example, both the skin incision and the skin excision schools favor making an incision to accurately define the placement of the crease. These practitioners are comfortable with these techniques as well as the wound healing process, and are likely to be less concerned about instant recovery. Specialists who routinely open the orbital septum are likewise comfortable with the anatomic landmarks and aim to clear the preaponeurotic zone along the superior tarsal border. Overall, the proponents of the external incision feel more comfortable with the predictability and permanence of this approach, and aim for a longer-lasting crease and less need for interval adjustment procedures. This approach, especially when carried out without the need for buried sutures, frequently yields a crease form that is subjectively comfortable for the patient on upgaze and downgaze, without the often-voiced complaint of tightness of the upper lid and a sensation of the buried sutures poking the pretarsal zone. The surgeon who operates through a 5–8 mm skin incision may be able to accomplish limited debulking of soft tissues. One drawback may be a crease that appears better formed over the central skin incision than over the medial and lateral portions of the lid.

The choice of suture material varies greatly, as do the closure techniques applied in the external incision methods. The techniques for construction of the upper eyelid crease fall into two broad categories: skin–levator–skin (or skin–tarsus–skin) and levator aponeurosis to inferior subcutaneous plane (or superior tarsal border to inferior subcutaneous plane: STB/inf.subQ).

Skin–Levator–Skin Approach

In this approach, sutures are placed so that the first bite is into the inferior skin edge, the second is into the dis-

tal fibers of the levator aponeurosis along the superior tarsal border, and the third is into the upper skin edge (Fig. 6-1). This maneuver allows an adhesion to form between the levator aponeurosis and the subdermal area along the superior tarsal border, closely approximating the distal interdigitations of the levator aponeurosis. Fernandez[1] wrote that this technique gives a 'dynamic' and superficial crease (Fig. 6-2), in contrast to the skin–tarsus–skin method, which tends to give a 'static' crease (Fig. 6-3).

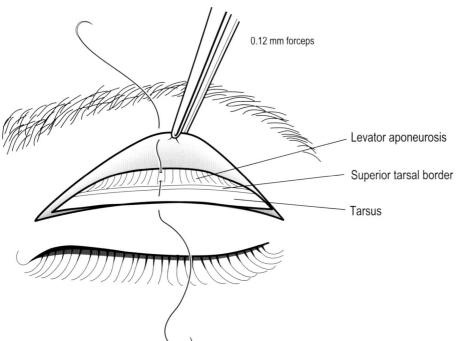

0.12 mm forceps

Levator aponeurosis

Superior tarsal border

Tarsus

Fig. 6-1 Skin–levator–skin closure. The stitch first passes through the lower skin border, taking a bite into the levator aponeurosis along the superior tarsal border (STB), and then through the upper skin border.

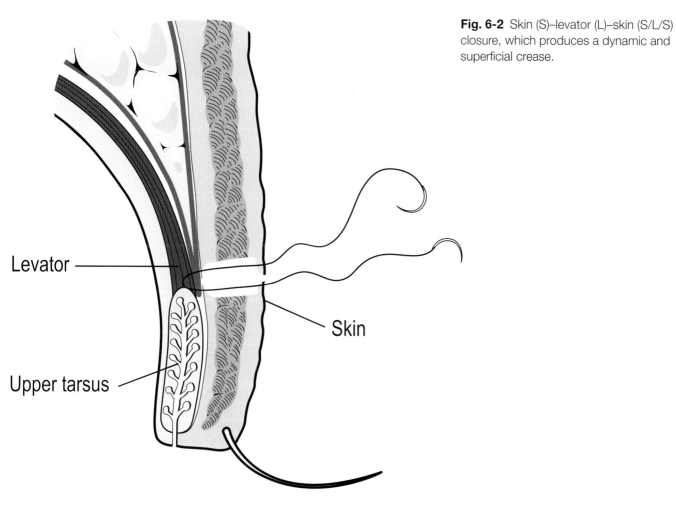

Fig. 6-2 Skin (S)–levator (L)–skin (S/L/S) closure, which produces a dynamic and superficial crease.

Levator

Upper tarsus

Skin

Suture passage from: Skin → Levator → Skin

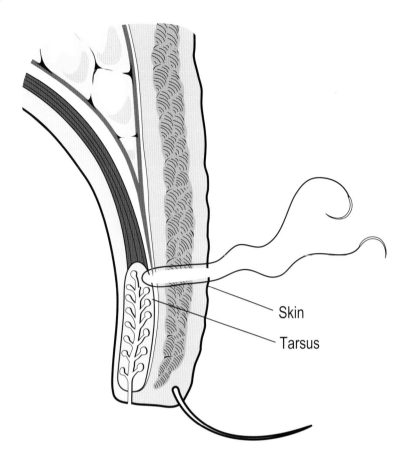

Fig. 6-3 Skin (S)–tarsus (T)–skin (S/T/S) closure, which tends to produce a static crease.

Skin

Tarsus

Suture passage from: Skin ➔ Tarsus ➔ Skin

Levator Aponeurosis to Inferior Subcutaneous Plane Approach

In the levator aponeurosis to inferior subcutaneous plane approach, several buried 6/0 nylon, polyglycolic acid, or polypropylene sutures are applied to allow adhesions to form between the levator aponeurosis and the subcutaneous tissue of the inferior incision along the superior tarsal border (Fig. 6-4). According to Fernandez,[1] this procedure also produces a dynamic crease, but a more deep and permanent one than in the skin–levator–skin method of closure. In 1974 and 1977, Sheen[2,3] described performing this technique on Caucasian patients who underwent upper blepharoplasty. Sutures were applied from the levator aponeurosis to the inferior orbicularis muscle (in essence the

inferior subcutaneous tissue). In 1976, Putterman and Urist,[4] and Weingarten[5] described the technique of applying sutures from the superior tarsal border to the inferior subcutaneous plane (Fig. 6-5).

In 1999 Park[6] published his technique of orbicularis–levator fixation in double-eyelid procedures for Asians. He used three 6/0 nylon sutures to fix a folded portion of the levator aponeurosis to the orbicularis oculi of the inferior skin edge.

Yoo[7] described crease formation simply by trimming of pretarsal fat and the placement of 'basting sutures' that eliminate the dead space formed by removal of pretarsal tissues, but without attaching any aponeurosis or tarsal plate. The author assumed that the reduction of the soft tissue between levator and skin was a more important factor in the formation of a crease than levator insertion to the skin. He advocated an open

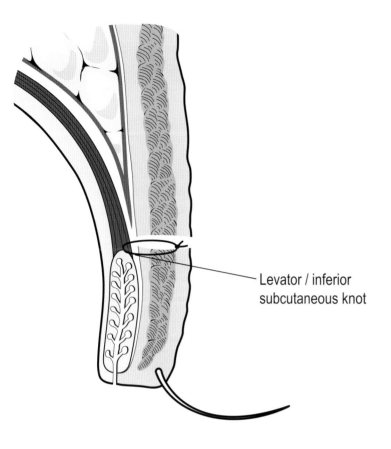

Fig. 6-4 Placement of ligature buried between the inferior subcutaneous tissues and the levator aponeurosis. According to Fernandez[1] this procedure results in a deeper and more permanent dynamic crease.

Levator / inferior
subcutaneous knot

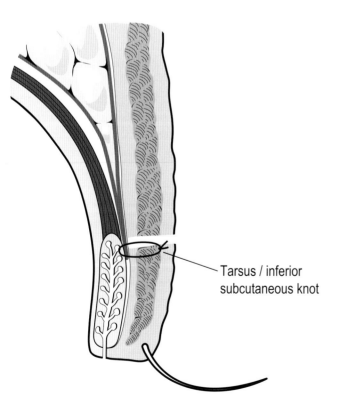

Fig. 6-5 Placement of ligature buried between tarsus and subcutaneous tissues of inferior skin edge.

Tarsus / inferior
subcutaneous knot

incisional method using removal of excessive soft tissue and closure without supratarsal fixation. He used a continuous 6/0 silk and three interrupted sutures to close the wound. Conceptually the three interrupted basting sutures were used to close the skin, orbicularis, and pretarsal soft tissues; however, the exact function of these interrupted sutures is debatable, as the closure of the dead space implied by the author following the removal of soft tissue will inherently anastomose the upper and lower skin margins together and over the levator aponeurosis along the superior tarsal margin. The net result would also be a rigid pretarsal platform allowing crease formation, and there would very likely be secondarily induced aponeurotic adhesions to the pretarsal tissues after such a maneuver. In addition, there is still the presence of other impeding factors, such as tissue redundancy in the preaponeurotic space above this region, which consists of the preseptal orbicularis, suborbicularis fat and septum as well as inferiorly migrated preaponeurotic fat pads. In Yoo's series of 48 patients, some appeared to show significant regression of the height of the crease after 1–2 years.

Lee et al.[8] advocated attachment of the orbital septum to the skin to form the eyelid crease. They stated that there are distinct layers of fascia anterior to the orbital septum that originate from the septum and insert on to the pretarsal aponeurotic expansion. Seeing that the preaponeurotic fat and orbital septum hang below the fusion line of the orbital septum and aponeurosis in Asian single eyelids, the authors advocated the septodermal fixation technique, where the hanging portion of the orbital septum is dissected from the aponeurosis, plicated, and then sutured to the skin of the pretarsal flap. The septum is not routinely opened, but the redundant portion hanging below the fusion line is sutured to the pretarsal skin–muscle flap. In 60% of their patients the pretarsal fibrofatty layers are removed to promote adhesion between the pretarsal orbicularis fascia and the pretarsal aponeurotic expansion. The authors followed 512 patients over 3 years, and the advantages they claim include less postoperative edema, less discomfort and pain, and satisfactory crease formation.

At the opposite end of the spectrum, in 1993 Flowers[9] described his approach towards upper blepharoplasty and crease fixation in Caucasians and Asians, utilizing his approach of 'anchor blepharoplasty'. He discussed the challenge when a crease fold was allowed to remain in an upper blepharoplasty – the pretarsal skin appeared excessive and wrinkled. His solution was to correlate the amount of pretarsal skin that is allowed to remain (the location of the lid incision) with the tarsal height, excising the desired skin with its supratarsal crease and then recreating a new precise crease fold by attaching the dermis of the pretarsal skin flap to the aponeurosis and tarsus.

The tarsus is everted and its height measured. It is marked on the skin side with the same distance from the lash line, which adds 2 mm to the distance as measured from the actual lid margin. Flowers' operative rule is that there should be 26–30 mm of skin on the upper lid between the eyebrow and the lid margin for normal contour and invagination as well as for closure. This is broken down into approximately 10 mm for the invagination of the eyelid fold, a minimum of 12 mm from the eyelid fold to the brow, and 3–6 mm of visible pretarsal skin; 1–2 mm are allowed for the curvature of the lid fold as it bends into the crease. If the amount is less than 26–30 mm there will be problems with invagination of the fold, as well as a restricted brow position and inadequate lid closure owing to shortage of skin. The amount of eyelid skin that overhangs and obstructs the desired view of the pretarsal skin is measured using a caliper, or estimated visually; this is doubled (×2) to arrive at the amount of skin that ought to be removed. This may be performed at different points along the eyelid. Flowers discussed the treatment of fat and its partial excision over the lateral quadrant, and the possibility of rotating and translocating the fat on to the medial aspect of the supratarsal sulcus. He believed that trimming pretarsal connective tissues and thinning of the pretarsal orbicularis on the underside of the pretarsal skin flap helps both to reduce postoperative edema in that region and to produce a smooth pretarsal skin surface as a result of adherence of the skin and orbicularis to the tarsus.

In this approach the plane between the pretarsal orbicularis and the distal insertion of the levator aponeurosis over the anterior surface of the upper tarsus is separated with scissors down to the lash margin. Any inferior attachment of the aponeurotic fibers to the skin is thus transected. The filmy pretarsal connective tissues, including portions of pretarsal orbicularis that may be excessive, are excised with scissors over the anterior tarsal surface. The dermis of the pretarsal skin

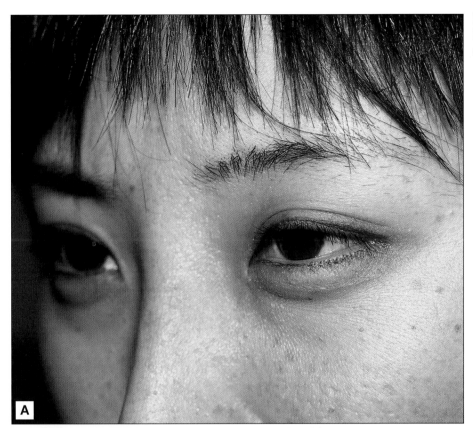

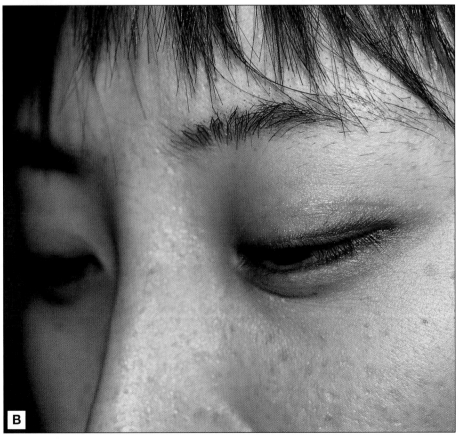

Fig. 6-6 (A) A dynamic crease is apparent on forward gaze but disappears on downgaze **(B)**.

flap (lower skin edge) is sutured subcuticularly to the superior margin of the tarsus as well as the free terminal edge of the aponeurosis using absorbable 6/0 Vicryl. Flowers usually applies three or four of these sutures centrally, and one or two laterally as well as medially along the new crease. (The trimming of the pretarsal tissues and excision of some of the anterior portion of the distal levator aponeurosis will invariably leave behind a free edge; this does not mean that the levator aponeurosis has been entirely transected.) In addition, the upper and lower skin edges are closed with a running non-dissolving suture, incorporating the aponeurosis in each bite.

Alternative methods of closure mentioned by Flowers were:

1. To use interrupted nylon sutures alone, incorporating all layers together: the lower skin edge, the superior tarsal border, the free edge of the aponeurosis, and the upper skin edge. No Vicryl is then used for the skin–tarsus–levator aponeurosis alone.
2. The incorporation of the upper and lower skin edges into the deeper 6/0 Vicryl that binds the superior tarsal border as well as the free edge of the aponeurosis. No nylon or non-dissolving suture is then used.

The reason for incorporating the levator aponeurosis, according to Flowers, is that it exerts a small amount of tension on the pretarsal skin and thereby keeps it taut. By the same reasoning, he anchors the pretarsal skin flap to the tarsus to prevent excessive pull by the aponeurosis on the pretarsal skin, resulting in eyelash eversion and excessive showing of the upper lid margin itself. The author stated that patients often experience some degree of ptosis, as well as a tugging feeling on upgaze. He stated that complete recovery requires 2–3 years, but that patients generally look very satisfactory by 2 weeks after surgery.

The concept of a dynamic versus a static crease is worth elaborating. When a person has a natural crease in the upper eyelid, the crease is well defined when that person looks straight ahead (Fig. 6-6A). On downgaze, the inferior rectus and superior oblique muscles contract, whereas the superior rectus, levator, and inferior oblique muscles relax. As the eyes look downward, the

upper lid follows and the upper lid crease loses prominence, sometimes becoming barely observable (Fig. 6-6B). A crease that is present when the levator is active and which fades from view when the levator relaxes is called a dynamic crease.

A surgically formed upper lid crease that is present and noticeable even on downgaze (when the levator is relaxed) is called a static crease. This type of crease is often seen in patients who have had the inferior skin edge sutured to the superior tarsal border and upper skin edge.

In practice the matter is not always predictable: a static crease is not always seen as a result of skin–tarsus–skin closure, and a dynamic crease does not always occur when skin–levator–skin or levator aponeurosis–inferior subcutaneous plane closure is performed.

This author[10–13] prefers the external incision method because it is more controlled and permanent. I remove a variable amount of skin depending on the patient's needs. I also resect some orbicularis oculi – usually several millimeters along the preseptal and the pretarsal segments. The orbital septum is opened superiorly and, depending on the situation, a variable amount of preaponeurotic fat may be trimmed, but never completely removed. The lid crease-enhancing sutures are placed skin–levator aponeurosis–skin. To give a dynamic, superficial crease I use non-absorbable non-reactive suture materials that are then removed. I do not use any buried suture materials.

References

1. Fernandez LR. Double eyelid operation in the Oriental in Hawaii. Plast Reconstruct Surg 1960;25:256–264.
2. Sheen JH. Supratarsal fixation in upper blepharoplasty. Plast Reconstruct Surg 1974;54:424–431.
3. Sheen JH. A change in the technique of supratarsal fixation in upper blepharoplasty. Plast Reconstruct Surg 1977;59:831–834.
4. Putterman AM, Urist MJ. Reconstruction of the upper eyelid crease and fold. Arch Ophthalmol 1976;94:1941–1954.

5. Weingarten CZ. Blepharoplasty in the oriental eye. Trans Am Acad Ophthalmol Otol 1976;82:442–446.

6. Park JI. Orbicularis–levator fixation in double-eyelid operation. Arch Facial Plast Surg 1999;1:90–95.

7. Yoo H-B. The double eyelid operation without supratarsal fixation. Plast Reconstruct Surg 1991;88:12–17.

8. Lee JS, Park WJ, Shin MS, Song IC. Simplified anatomic method of double-eyelid operation: septodermal fixation technique. Plast Reconstruct Surg 1997;100:170–178.

9. Flowers RS. Upper blepharoplasty by eyelid invagination – anchor blepharoplasty. Clin Plast Surg 1993;20:193–207.

10. Chen WPD. Asian blepharoplasty. Ophthalm Plast Reconstruct Surg 1987;3:135–140.

11. Chen WPD. A comparison of Caucasian and Asian blepharoplasty. Ophthalm Pract 1991;9:216–222.

12. Chen WPD. Upper blepharoplasty in the Asian patient. In: Putterman AM, ed. Cosmetic oculoplastic surgery, 3rd edn. Philadelphia: WB Saunders, 2000: Chapter 11.

13. Chen WPD, Khan J, McCord CD Jr. Color atlas of cosmetic oculofacial surgery. Oxford: Butterworth–Heinemann, 2004.

Asian Blepharoplasty Steps: The First Vector

Chapter 7

William P.D. Chen

When trying to achieve the optimal placement of a lid crease with the proper height, shape, continuity and permanence, a modified external incision technique allows maximum control. The following steps will be discussed in detail over the next two chapters: premedication and surgical setup; the anesthetic mixture and injections; and surgical steps – marking of the crease, skin incision and skin excision.

- The first vector – bevelled surgical plane and opening of orbital septum;
- The second vector – excision of orbicularis and septum as a preaponeurotic platform along the superior tarsal border (Chapter 8):
  - optional excision of the preaponeurotic fat pads;
  - excision of a strip of inferior pretarsal orbicularis;
  - formation of the lid crease;
  - closure of the wound.

Premedication and Surgical Preparation

The patient usually receives 10 mg of diazepam and 5 mg of Vicodin orally 60–90 minutes before the procedure. They are then placed in the supine position, and an intravenous line and electrocardiograph monitors are applied. A pulse oximeter that provides a real-time readout of the patient's PaO_2 is applied. A nasal cannula is applied to administer 2 L/min room air.

Anesthetic Mixture and Injections

I prepare two mixtures of local anesthetic. First, I draw up 10 mL of 2% lidocaine (Xylocaine) containing 1:100 000 dilution of epinephrine (this is an acidic mixture and is labeled 'Regular'). In areas where hyaluronidase is available, the use of 150 units mixed into the 10 mL of the above mixture is helpful. Second, 1 mL of 2% xylocaine is further diluted with 9 mL of injectable normal saline. This mixture now has a pH closer to neutrality, as it has been diluted with the buffering action of injectable normal saline. The epinephrine concentration is now 1:1 000 000 (labeled 'Diluted').

I apply a drop of topical anesthetic, 0.5% proparacaine hydrochloride, on each eye for comfort prior to surgical preparation and draping. Using a 30 gauge needle I infiltrate 0.25–0.5 mL of the diluted anesthetic subcutaneously along the superior tarsal border (Fig. 7-1).

During the next few minutes the anesthetic takes effect and one can observe blanching of the eyelid skin owing to the powerful vasoconstrictive effect of the diluted epinephrine–anesthetic mixture (Fig. 7-2).

I then inject the regular 2% xylocaine with epinephrine in the suborbicularis plane along the superior tarsal border, usually giving less than 0.75 mL per lid.

The purpose of this two-stage injection is to allow for a relatively painless preinfiltration to anesthetize the surgical field before the full strength of acidic 2% xylocaine is given.[1] (One may add sodium bicarbonate to the 2% mixture to achieve the same effect: for a 10% volume mixture, 1 mL of 8.4% sodium bicarbonate containing 8.4 g or 100 mEq/100 mL is mixed with 9 mL of the 2% xylocaine.) If hyaluronidase is available it may be used, and the enzyme promotes dispersion of the anesthetic and greatly reduces any tissue distortion, thereby facilitating the identification of any crease line the patient may have.

When confronted with a patient with a low pain threshold one may supplement the local field infiltration with a frontal nerve block. A 30 gauge half-inch needle may be used to apply 0.5 mL of the anesthetic into the supraorbital space just lateral to the supraorbital notch.

The eyelids and face are then prepared and cleansed in the usual fashion for ophthalmic plastic surgery. The eyes again receive a drop of topical anesthetic, this time using tetracaine hydrochloride for longer-lasting corneal anesthesia. To eliminate the sensation of claustrophobia that often occurs with full draping over the nose and midface, room air is delivered through a nasal cannula. Opaque black corneal protectors are then applied over each eye.

Skin Blanching Following Injection of Diluted Xylocaine with Epinephrine

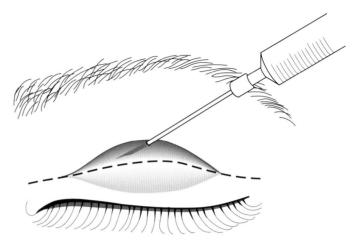

Fig. 7-1 Initial subcutaneous injection of diluted, pH-balanced anesthetic mixture.

 Pearls for this step:

1. The use of a diluted anesthetic solution helps to reduce the pain of injection, reduce the volume of anesthetic needed for injection, and reduce tissue distortion as a result of less volume expansion and reduced bleeding. It allows the surgeon to stay focused on the surgical plane.

2. The use of nasally delivered room air or low-flow oxygen serves to lessen the patient's sense of claustrophobia.

 Pitfalls:

1. Never use nasal oxygen in an open system exposed to monopolar cautery as it may cause ignition and flaming.

2. Always apply pulse oximetry to measure the Pao_2 saturation. Preoperative and intraoperative sedation may easily cause apnea in a sensitive patient.

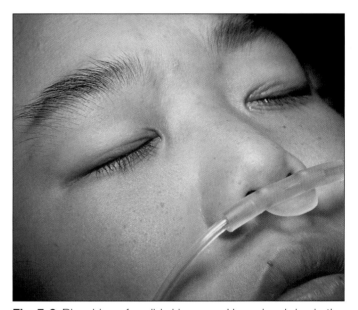

Fig. 7-2 Blanching of eyelid skin caused by epinephrine in the anesthetic mixture.

Eversion of Tarsus and Measurement of Tarsal Height Using a Caliper (Fig. 7-3)

The height of the tarsus determines the overall central position of the surgical crease; the shape is determined by the medial and lateral thirds of this lower line of incision, designed according to the patient's preference.

The shaved-off tip of a cotton-tipped wooden applicator dipped in methylene blue is used to mark the proposed crease. The upper lid is everted and the vertical height of the tarsus measured over the central portion of the lid with a caliper. This measurement is usually between 6.5 and 7.5 mm. It is carefully transcribed on to the external skin surface, again over the central part of the eyelid skin. This point directly overlies the superior tarsal border and will serve as a reference point for the overall crease *height* along the *central* one-third of the eyelid, whether the crease *shape* is to be nasally tapered, parallel, or laterally flared (rare). For those patients who have a crease, one should also measure the tarsus to confirm that the apparent crease is indeed the correct line to use, whether one is planning to preserve it or enhance it.

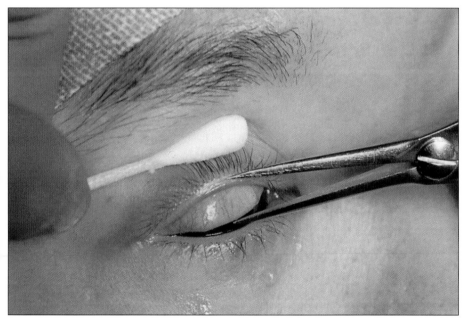

Fig. 7-3 The upper lid is everted and the tarsal height is measured over the central portion.

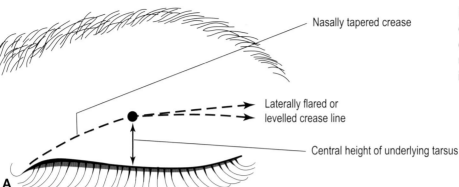

Nasally tapered crease

Laterally flared or
levelled crease line

Central height of underlying tarsus

A

Fig. 7-4 (A) Design of a nasally tapered crease. The lateral portion may be designed to be level or flared slightly upward. **(B)** The nasally tapered crease is marked; the lateral portion is leveled.

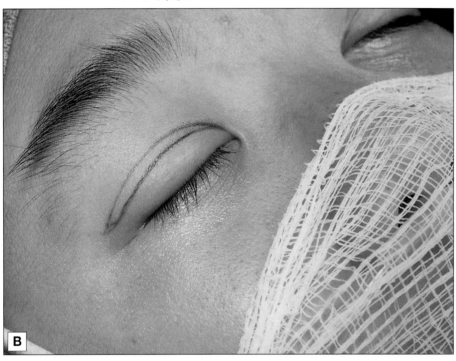

B

Design of the Nasally Tapered Crease and Marking (Fig. 7-4)

If the crease is to be nasally tapered, with either a laterally leveled or a flared configuration, the *medial* one-third of the incision line is marked such that it tapers towards the medial canthal angle or merges with the medial upper lid fold. The *lateral* one-third is usually marked in a level configuration, although occasionally a patient may request a slight upward widening over the lateral segment of the crease.

 Pearls for this step:

■ The use of the tapered tip of a wooden stick dipped in ink or dye allows precise drawing and redrawing, compared to the usual marking pen available in operating theaters.

 Pearls for this step:

■ In Asian blepharoplasty involving skin excision, the lower incision line will determine the height and shape of the surgically created crease.

■ Repetitive measurements and confirmation of incision lines are important.

■ Usually 1–3 mm of skin is included in the incision line for excision.

■ Using the thinned wooden applicator to physically apply very gentle pressure on the lower incision line (proposed line for new crease formation), instruct the patient to look upwards before the incision starts in order to simulate and assess how the crease may appear. Because the eyelid has been injected, the crease will appear more swollen and further from the ciliary margin than postoperatively, after it is eventually healed.

Design of the Parallel Crease and Marking (Fig. 7-5)

For a parallel crease, the measured height of the superior tarsal border is drawn across the width of the eyelid skin.

To recapitulate, the height of the tarsus determines the overall central position of the surgical crease; the shape is determined by how the medial and lateral thirds of this crease (lower line of incision) are designed, depending on the patient's preference.

To create adequate adhesions, it is necessary to remove some subdermal tissue. A strip of skin measuring approximately 2 mm is then marked above and parallel to the *lower* line of incision. In the patient who desires a nasally tapered configuration the *upper* line of incision is also tapered towards the medial canthal angle, or merged with any medial upper lid fold that may be present. This segment of skin to be excised is often less than 2 mm over the medial portion of the crease.

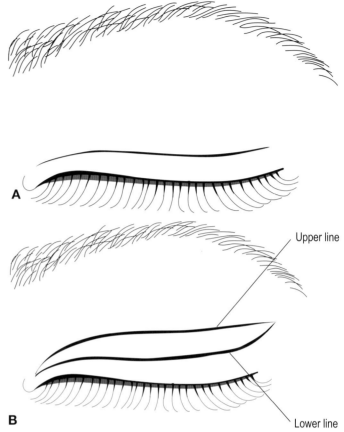

Upper line

Lower line

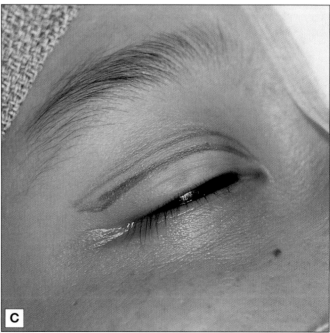

 Pearls for this step:

In designing the parallel crease there is an unconscious tendency to converge towards the medial canthal angle and thereby turn it into a nasally tapered crease. I often intentionally draw the tapering crease first and then use it as a visual guide to decide how a parallel crease should be designed near the medial third of the upper lid, to remind myself to stay parallel.

 Pitfalls:

■ Medially, the parallel crease does not flare upward from the medial canthal angle.

■ The medial end of the crease design should not go past an imaginary vertical line aligned with the medial canthal angle for both nasally tapered and parallel creases.

■ Laterally, the crease design should not traverse past the lateral canthal angle.

Fig. 7-5 (A) Design for a parallel crease. **(B)** Design for a parallel crease including the upper and lower lines of incision. **(C)** Nasally tapered crease with a lateral flare.

Skin Incision Along the Upper and Lower Lines of Incision (Fig. 7-6)

The incision is then carried out using a no.15 surgical blade (Bard–Parker) along the upper and lower lines, incising just through the dermis and barely within the superficial orbicularis oculi muscles. Fine capillary bleeding is controlled using a bipolar Wetfield cautery.

The excision of a strip of skin is not necessary in every case; however, it is the author's belief that it facilitates the removal of subsequent layers of lid tissue, thereby allowing adequate crease formation. At this point the superior tarsal border is still covered by pretarsal and supratarsal orbicularis oculi muscle, possibly with some terminal portions of the orbital septum, and the terminal fibers of the levator aponeurosis beneath the septum. (I prefer the term supratarsal to preseptal, as the supratarsal area is directly above the tarsus, whereas the true 'preseptal' region, implying an area in front of where orbital septum is present, may be quite a few millimeters superior to this, as the septum fuses to the aponeurosis a variable distance from the superior tarsal border.)

 Pearls for this step:

- It is important to stabilize the tarsal plate and overlying soft tissues and skin when making a continuous incision, especially along the lower line of incision; this is a critical step in the outcome of the designed crease.

- The continuous incision may be performed in three steps so that one may check and recheck the passage. For right-handed surgeons, for the right upper lid it is best to start medially, and for the left upper lid one may start from the lateral end of the incision line.

- Any bleeding is best controlled with bipolar cautery via a fine jeweler's tip. This allows the surgeon to reduce any immediate tissue swelling and obscuration of the tissue planes, thereby maintaining a clear operative field. Furthermore, it allows one to stay within the planned incision line.

 Pitfalls:

It is easy to incise too deeply and cause a small steady bleed from the orbicularis muscle, which will soon develop into a hematoma and distort the incision line as well as the incision planes, blurring the distinction between fat, orbicularis, orbital septum and levator aponeurosis along the superior tarsal border. This may occur de novo from the vascular orbicularis, or actually while traversing through one of the anastomotic branches between the marginal and peripheral arcades. It may result in transient postoperative secondary ptosis.

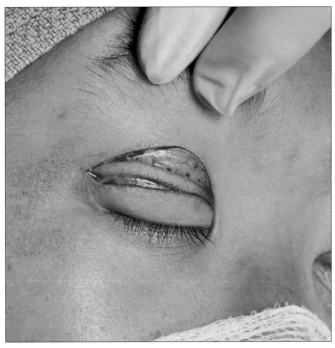

Fig. 7-6 The upper and lower incision lines have been made using a no.15 surgical blade.

First Vector: Beveled Transection Through the Orbicularis Muscle Along the Upper Incision Line and Opening of the Orbital Septum (Fig. 7-7)

At this point the superior tarsal border is still covered by pretarsal and preseptal orbicularis oculi muscle, the terminal portions of the orbital septum, and the anteriorly directed terminal fibers of the levator aponeurosis beneath the septum.

One may use the fingers of the left hand to retract the upper incision wound edge slightly, then aim a bovie cautery tip (or a radiofrequency unit's Empire tip needle) superiorly to transect through the preseptal orbicularis oculi in an oblique fashion, knowing that although the upper incision line is only 2–3 mm above the superior tarsal border, with the upward beveling the bovie tip is aiming at a point above where the septum fuses with the aponeurosis. (In Asians, the orbital septum may join the aponeurosis as low as 2–3 mm above the superior tarsal border.) The cutting cautery tip is used in a feather-light fashion so as to reach the orbital septum gently. There may be some preseptal fat. When the septum over the central one-third is opened, one can see the slightly bulging preaponeurotic fat pad prolapsing through the opening. A blunt-tipped

Westcott's spring scissors is then used to open the orbital septum along the superior line of incision, and the skin–orbicularis–orbital septum flap is turned inferiorly along the superior tarsal border.

Pearls for this step:

Always tilt the tips of the scissors upward when extending the horizontal release of the orbital septum to either side. The purpose is to avoid inadvertent injury to the vessels within the fat pad, the fat pad itself, the underlying levator aponeurosis, or the lobe of the lacrimal gland situated over the lateral end.

Pitfalls:

- In opening the orbital septum medially, the levator aponeurosis may be injured.

- In opening of the lateral extent of the septum, the lacrimal gland can be injured.

- Avoid the use of monopolar cautery over the superior medial aspect of the orbital space to avoid the trochlea of the superior oblique muscle, which can lead to fourth nerve palsy and torsional diplopia.

- Avoid cauterizing the lacrimal gland over the superior lateral aspect of the anterior orbital rim.

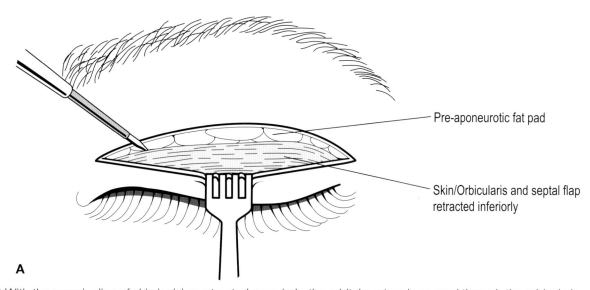

Pre-aponeurotic fat pad

Skin/Orbicularis and septal flap retracted inferiorly

A

Fig. 7-7 **(A)** With the superior line of skin incision retracted superiorly, the orbital septum is opened through the orbicularis muscle with a monopolar cautery tip at the lowest setting of cutting mode.

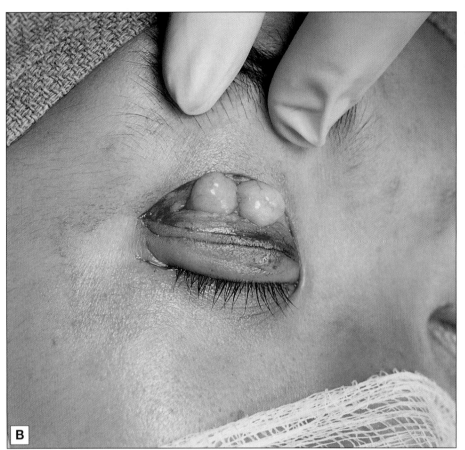

Fig. 7-7 (B) The orbital septum is opened along the superior line of incision. Preaponeurotic fat pads can be seen from where the septum is opened.

Reference

1. Tenzel RR, Hustead RF, Schietroma J, Hustead J. The best trick I learned this year. Presented at the Annual Scientific Symposium of the American Society of Ophthalmic Plastic and Reconstructive Surgery, New Orleans, 1986.

William P.D. Chen

Rotation and Teasing of Myocutaneous Strip away from the Underlying Levator Aponeurosis and Preaponeurotic Fat Pad, Hinging It along the Superior Tarsal Border. Also Shows Preaponeurotic Fat Being Separated from the Underlying Levator

A Westcott scissors is used to open the potential space between the preaponeurotic fat and the overlying orbic-ularis muscle within the redundant myocutaneous strip, retracting it with a Blair's tissue retractor (Fig. 8-1A). The central preaponeurotic fat pad is dissected and separated from its fascial attachment to its underly-ing levator muscle fibers (Fig. 8-1B) (the levator is salmon-colored, with vertically oriented muscle stria-tions). The fat should be repositioned and allowed to fill in the space between the levator and the anterior aspect of the superior orbital rim (the supratarsal sulcus).

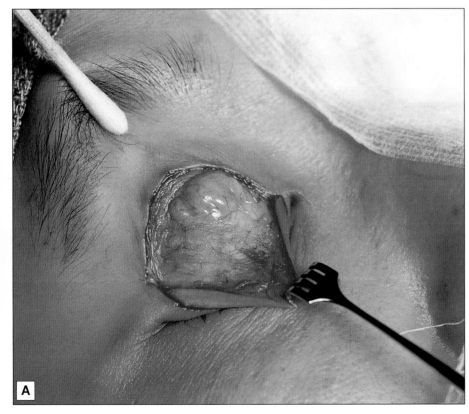

Fig. 8-1 (A) The skin–orbicularis–orbital septum flap is retracted inferiorly using a tissue retractor, allowing access to the preaponeurotic fat pad (right upper lid).

A

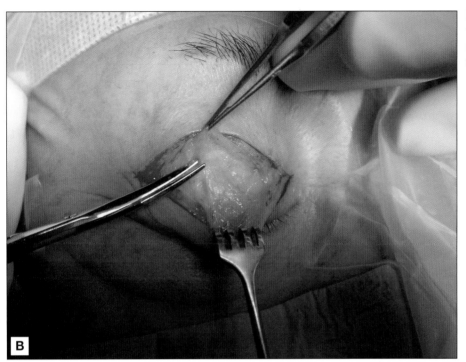

Fig. 8-1 (B) Dissection and elevation of the preaponeurotic fat pad from the underlying levator aponeurosis (right upper lid).

Pearls for this step:

■ After separating the initial fine adhesions of fat from the overlying orbicularis, it is often safer to use moist cotton-tipped applicators to separate the fat from the underlying superior tarsal border, levator aponeurosis, and levator muscle.

■ No attempt is made to remove fat pads unless they are grossly interfering with crease formation along the superior tarsal border; a Wetfield bipolar cautery may be used to shrink them away if they are potentially 'threatening' the optimal construction of the crease by their presence directly over the preaponeurotic platform.

Pitfalls:

■ Avoid pointing the scissors posteriorly towards the levator as you elevate the myocutaneous flap.

■ After the myocutaneous flap has been elevated, avoid cutting any fat that may be intertwined on the underbelly of the myocutaneous strip; this may cause bleeding of the intrafat blood vessels, as well as inadvertent reduction in the volume of preaponeurotic fat left behind.

Optional Excision of Preaponeurotic Fat Pad (Fig. 8-2)

Occasionally, in patients with very full upper lids, significant fat is seen both centrally and inferiorly. This may significantly abort/interfere with any attempt to form a crease. In these patients, instead of mild reduction with bipolar cautery one may opt to excise 25–50% of the preaponeurotic fat in the surgical field. A Wetfield cautery is used to treat the intrafat vessels first, then cutting monopolar cautery is used to cut the fat pad 2–3 mm at a time; these maneuvers are then repeated. It may take two to three repetitions before this step is complete. (The fat excision often requires a small supplement of lidocaine injection in the space underneath the preaponeurotic fat pad.)

If a patient with dermatochalasis and crease obliteration manifests even a very minimal concavity in the supratarsal sulcus, one should not remove any fat as this will worsen the hollowness and result in multiple redundant folds superior to where one wishes the crease to be. Instead of excising the fat, one should reposit it higher.

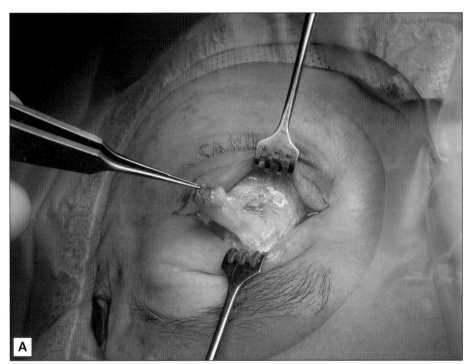

Fig. 8-2 (A) Partial excision of inferior portion of the preaponeurotic fat pad (left upper lid).

 Pearls for this step:

- Extra care and time are allotted to the reduction of fat pads, if elected. Hemorrhage from undetected bleeders following transection of the intrafat vessels may lead to serious consequences, including orbital hematoma and blindness.

- A prolapsed lacrimal gland may look like a lobe of fat. It must be recognized and needs to be reanchored to a point behind the superolateral orbital rim using an absorbable suture.

Pitfalls:

- It is important to clearly distinguish the nasal fat pad and the central preaponeurotic fat pad from the lacrimal gland lobule.

- Transection of the lacrimal gland may lead to varying degrees of dry eye.

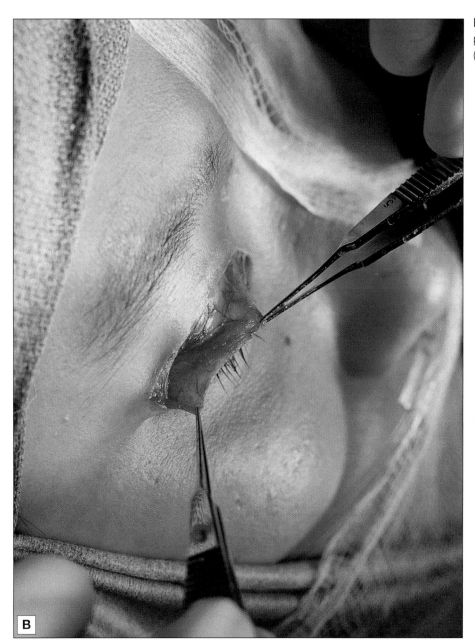

Fig. 8-2 (B) A very small amount of preaponeurotic fat pad may be excised (right upper lid).

B

Excision of the Myocutaneous Flap (Skin, Orbicularis, and Inferior Remnants of Orbital Septum) along the Superior Tarsal Border (Fig. 8-3)

This is carried out by grasping the lateral end of the myocutaneous flap of the right upper lid (or the medial end of the left upper lid myocutaneous flap) with the instrument in your left hand, then using the monopolar needle tip in cutting mode or the radiofrequency unit to cut along a plane between the orbicularis within the flap and the superior tarsal border/aponeurotic junction.

Pitfalls:

- One must take care to avoid inadvertent partial transection of the distal fibers of the levator aponeurosis.

- Avoid transection of the superior tarsal vascular arcade, which may bleed and cause segmental swelling and postoperative secondary ptosis.

Pearls for this step:

- When the myocutaneous flap is incised, the orbicularis muscle will bleed. As one proceeds one should control each new bleeder with the bipolar cautery as soon as it arises, rather than cutting off the whole strip before coming back to control a group of bleeders. In the author's view this seems to reduce postoperative edema and hematoma formation.

- There is a tendency to go too shallow over the medial starting point of the left upper lid during this phase of the excision of the myocutaneous strip, leaving behind too much orbicularis. An inadequately anchored crease over the medial segment may therefore result from this subtle oversight.

Fig. 8-3 The flap of skin, orbicularis muscle, and septum superior to the superior tarsal border is excised.

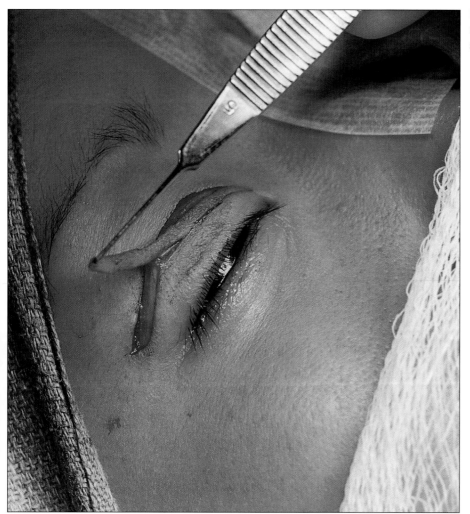

Further Discussion

The excision of a strip of skin is not necessary in every case; however, it is the author's belief that it facilitates the removal of subsequent layers of the lid tissue in order to form a good crease. The flap of myocutaneous and fascial tissues hinged along the superior tarsal border that is excised measures approximately 2–3 mm (Fig. 8-3).

In this situation the fragment of skin–orbicularis–septum that has been removed typically contains more orbicularis than skin, and so resembles a trapezoid in cross-sectional view, with the narrower of the two parallel planes being the external skin and the lengthier opposite side being the orbicularis with septum.

This second plane of transection (second vector) is performed perpendicular to the eyelid's skin surface and tracing along the lower line of skin incision (the future crease line).

The goal is to eliminate or thin the redundant fascial tissues in the preaponeurotic plane along the superior tarsal border. This platform of tissues may be termed the 'preaponeurotic platform', as it consists of all tissues anterior to the levator aponeurosis, and includes orbital septum, suborbicularis fat if any, preseptal orbicularis, subcutaneous fat (if any), and skin. This platform is removed in a uniform and equidepth fashion, conceptually as a trapezoidal block of tissues in cross-section.

This trapezoidal debulking involves only two vectors or two planes of tissue transection: the first is a beveled plane through the orbicularis until the orbital septum is reached, and the second is when the myocutaneous–septal flap is excised by transecting the orbicularis along the crease line. Bleeding can therefore occur only during these two steps, thereby minimizing the potential for crease irregularity and discrepancy in crease height during the immediate postoperative period.

If the skin, orbicularis, and septum are removed layer by layer, the extra steps involved (two with the skin: upper and lower incision lines; two with orbicularis; and two with the septum) may generate more bleeding there as well as from the interphase between the layers while removing them (skin-from-orbicularis, orbicularis-from-septum, and septum-from-levator). This multitude of possibilities for bleeding is simply unnecessary and is solved by utilizing this en-bloc trapezoidal debulking of the preaponeurotic platform.

There are 'intermediate' schools of the external incision methods in several noteworthy directions:

1. Some surgeons prefer to keep most of the septum intact and create just a single central opening through it to tease out the preaponeurotic fat for excision. A challenge one may encounter is that most preaponeurotic fat is located over the lateral half of the levator, and the excision of a portion of it without the benefit of a full view of its distribution may predispose to crease irregularity.

2. Some have proposed making a 5–8 mm skin incision at each of the three sites usually used in traditional suture ligation methods. Here again the orbital septum is then partially opened at each of the three locations and the fat selectively removed.

3. Some authors mention making a single 5–8 mm skin incision, and through an open septum then excising the preaponeurotic fat by pulling it centrally from the medial and lateral sectors. Crease fixation is then carried out as in any of the typical external incision methods. The supportive clinical photographs of this method appeared to show a much wider skin incision. One problem that may manifest with this approach is that the crease may be less well formed medially and laterally, and better formed centrally.

Pearls for this step:

- This trapezoidal 'one-plane' debulking of the preaponeurotic platform is an efficient, elegant and controlled technique of excising a whole block of redundant tissues, with full control of the tissues excised in an equi-depth fashion.

- The beveled plane allows the tissues to appose nicely during surgical closure.

- Instruct the patient to look up to evaluate your attempt at crease formation. Any incomplete crease formation should be investigated at this point.

Excision of Inferior Edge of Pretarsal Orbicularis Muscle (Fig. 8-4)

After the previous steps of excision of the myocutaneous strip, often there are some residual fascial tissues along the lower skin incision wound. This is composed of a combination of preseptal as well as pretarsal orbicularis muscle fibers, interspersed with an occasional pretarsal fat patch. This may occupy the path along which one is planning to form the crease just over the superior tarsal border. In this situation it is advisable to excise this 2–3 mm strip of orbicularis tissue along the inferior skin incision edge. It allows a slight flattening of the tissues along the pretarsal plane, as well as thinning of the inferior wound edge.

Some surgeons routinely debulk the entire pretarsal subcutaneous tissue, believing it is better to have only skin over the anterior surface of the tarsus. My experience differs, and I remove pretarsal tissue only if pretarsal fat is quite abundant and threatens the surgical formation of the desired upper lid crease. In the pretarsal plane of a creaseless Asian eyelid, there are few if any terminal interdigitations of the levator aponeurosis to the tissue beneath the dermis. I refrain from vigorous dissection along the pretarsal plane, because it leads to prolonged postoperative edema and can risk the undesirable sequela of the formation of more than one crease (Fig. 8-5). Furthermore, it is quite normal for Asians born with a natural crease to have some degree of pretarsal fullness along the area between the crease and the eyelashes (Fig. 8-6).

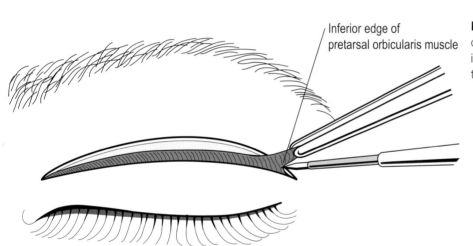

Inferior edge of pretarsal orbicularis muscle

Fig. 8-4 A small strip of pretarsal orbicularis muscle is trimmed along the inferior skin incision below the superior tarsal border.

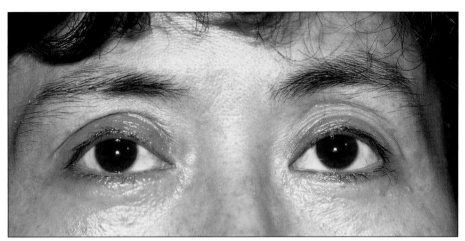

Fig. 8-5 Asian patient who underwent blepharoplasty. A hollow sulcus and the formation of multiple creases has occurred over both pretarsal and preseptal regions. Note the presence of a bifid crease over the medial portion of the right upper lid.

Pearls for this step:

■ The pretarsal tissue may be reduced only if pretarsal fat is moderately abundant and threatens the surgical formation of the desired upper lid crease.

■ There are some authors who routinely debulk the entire pretarsal subcutaneous tissue, believing that it is better to have only skin over the anterior surface of the tarsus. This may come about because of concerns that there are competing distal fibers of the levator aponeurosis within the pretarsal plane. In fact, within the pretarsal plane of a creaseless Asian eyelid there are few if any functional terminal interdigitations of the levator aponeurosis to the dermis.

Pitfalls:

■ Vigorous dissection along the pretarsal plane is not advisable as it creates prolonged postoperative edema and can risk the undesirable formation of multiple creases.

■ Leaving behind redundant tissues along the inferior border may result in only partial formation of the crease, or late obliteration of an initially acceptable crease.

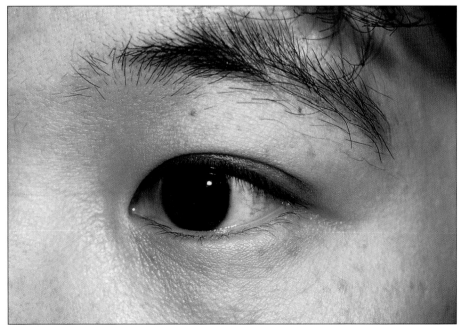

Fig. 8-6 A natural Asian crease showing some pretarsal fullness.

Wound Closure and Crease Formation (Fig. 8-7)

The adhesive surgical drapes over the patient's mid-forehead and upper eyelid skin are loosened to reduce any upward traction over the incision wound, tarsus, and eyelid margin. The forehead, brow and upper lid has been re-set.

In order to form a dynamic crease, the terminal fibers of the levator aponeurosis above the superior tarsal border should be directed to the subdermal plane of the lower line of skin incision. Non-absorbable sutures of 6/0 silk or nylon are used to pick up the lower skin edge and subcutaneous tissue, the levator aponeurosis along the superior tarsal border, and then the upper skin edge. Each of these is tied as an interrupted suture (Fig. 8-7A).

Besides the stitch over the center of the crease, three interrupted sutures are placed medially and two or three laterally (Fig. 8-7B and D). With these crease-forming sutures in place, the rest of the incision may

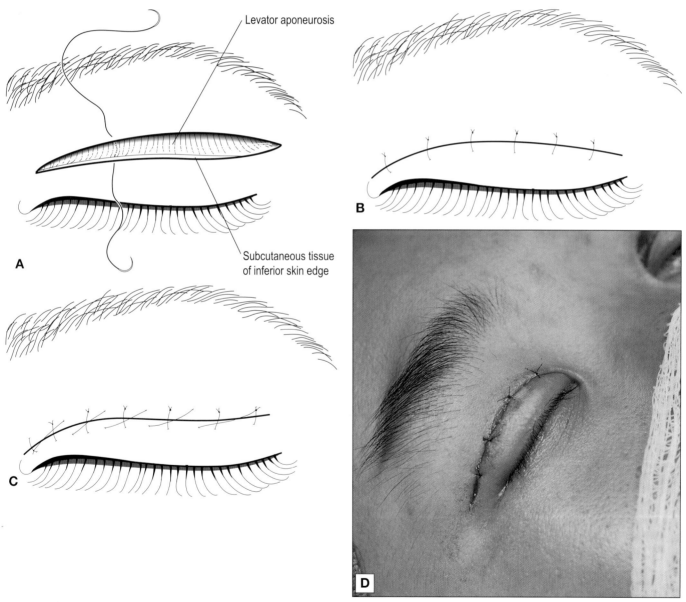

Fig. 8-7 (A) Skin–levator–skin closure along the superior tarsal border. **(B)** Use of five to six skin–levator–skin stitches. **(C)** Use of a single continuous suture over the wound edges. **(D)** Right upper lid wound closure following placement of four skin-levator-skin stitches.

be closed using 6/0 or 7/0 silk/nylon in a continuous or subcuticular fashion (Fig. 8-7C). This gives the best chance of forming a dynamic crease. (A dynamic crease of the upper eyelid is a surgically created crease that fades on downgaze. A static crease remains obvious on downgaze.)

Some surgeons prefer to bury either dissolvable or permanent stitches along the superior tarsal border, fixing the inferior edge of the pretarsal orbicularis to the levator muscle. In the author's experience, however, this method tends to create a static crease. Some patients complain of a persistent 'foreign body' sensation within the muscle layers of the lid many years after buried permanent sutures were applied. These often had to be removed secondarily.

Pearls for this step:

- The medial end of the crease may require the placement of additional crease-forming (skin–levator–skin) sutures, as the medial extent of the levator muscle is often rudimentary and underdeveloped.

- In a patient with medial canthal fold, if a nasally tapered crease shape has been selected the crease line can often be designed to merge medially into the fold itself.

- In applying the crease-forming stitch, each bite on the aponeurosis should be at the superior tarsal border and no higher, to prevent the formation of a 'high, harsh and semilunar crease'.

- To enhance or deepen a crease, one may apply three double-armed 5/0 Vicryl sutures transcutaneously to the underlying tarsus along the superior tarsal border (locating them over the medial, central, and lateral thirds of the eyelid) just below the crease line, in addition to the skin closure (Fig. 8-8). The sutures are then tied externally. After 1 week the knot is trimmed off the skin, leaving behind the buried loop of absorbable Vicryl.

- Check the symmetry of the crease bilaterally upon completion of closure. Measure the crease height with a caliper. If there is a discrepancy, it is better to correct the difference between the two sides by revising the higher crease downwards by excising 0.5–1 mm of skin from the inferior edge of this side. This is a general rule and should be applied only with individual evaluation.

Pitfalls:

- One is likely to end up with upper eyelid retraction or secondary ectropion if the tissues have not been allowed to lie back in their natural plane prior to surgical closure.

- Insufficient inclusion of the levator aponeurosis will result in partial crease formation or late obliteration.

- Excessively deep or high bites along the levator aponeurosis may result in a high crease or an acquired secondary ptosis, with secondary lagophthalmos on upgaze.

- Patients who manifest ptosis will tend to have poor crease formation. It is best to address the ptosis repair first, and return later to create a crease.

- The inclusion of residual fat pads along the superior tarsal border will result in obliteration of the crease.

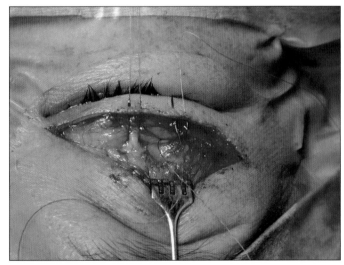

Fig. 8-8 Application of transcutaneous skin–tarsus fixation sutures along the lower skin edge.

Advanced Technique

For some patients it may be desirable to provide a crease that is not only dynamic and superficial but also lightly folded in when seen in the full frontal view. To achieve this, I have tried to leave some overlying strands of pretarsal and preseptal orbicularis muscle along the superior tarsal border and then close the wound by going skin–aponeurosis–skin. One can also vary the degree of levator aponeurotic attachment to the crease by varying the depth of the needle as it passes through the aponeurosis.

Solutions for Elderly Asian Patients

Elderly Asian patients, with or without a prior upper lid crease, may present with dermatochalasis alone (Fig. 8-9), dermatochalasis with fatty prolapse, or dermatochalasis with ptosis (Fig. 8-10).

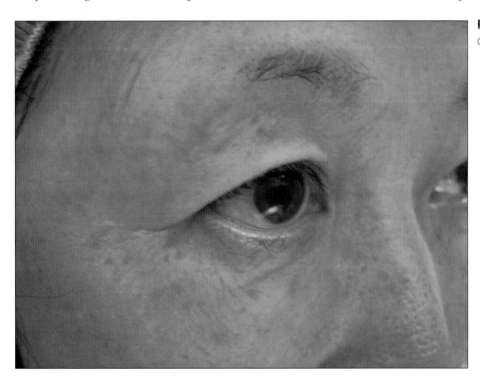

Fig. 8-9 Elderly Asian eyelid with dermatochalasis.

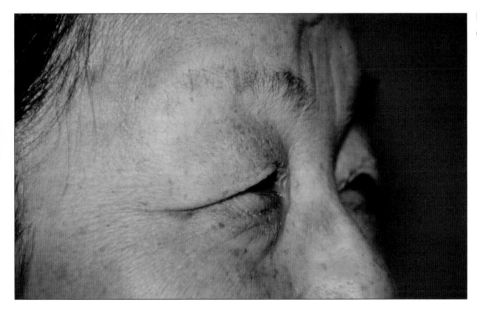

Fig. 8-10 Asian eyelid with dermatochalasis and involutional ptosis.

The surgical solutions for an elderly Asian patient with a pre-existing crease are as follows (Fig. 8-11):

1. Dermatochalasis alone is corrected by preserving the crease and performing a skin-excision blepharoplasty.
2. Dermatochalasis with fatty prolapse is best managed by preserving the crease and performing a blepharoplasty with trimming of only sufficient fat above the superior tarsal border to allow preservation of the crease (excess fat excision will result in deepening of the supratarsal sulcus).
3. In dermatochalasis with ptosis the crease has often migrated upward; it should be reset based on the individual's tarsal height using Asian blepharoplasty, performing only skin excision plus levator aponeurotic repair (resection and/or advancement).

When an elderly Asian patient does not have a pre-existing crease they have the option of having a crease added:

1. Dermatochalasis alone is corrected by Asian blepharoplasty with excision of the dermatochalasis and the creation of a crease.
2. Dermatochalasis with fatty prolapse is corrected by Asian blepharoplasty with excision of the dermatochalasis and the creation of a crease, with trimming of just sufficient fat to allow this.
3. Dermatochalasis with ptosis is corrected by skin excision-only Asian blepharoplasty and the creation of a crease, plus levator aponeurosis repair (resection and/or advancement).

When the elderly Asian patient does not have a pre-existing crease and prefers to remain crease free:

1. Dermatochalasis alone is corrected by skin excision blepharoplasty and closure without crease creation.
2. Dermatochalasis with fatty prolapse is corrected by skin excision blepharoplasty, minimal fat excision, and closure without crease creation.
3. Dermatochalasis with ptosis is corrected by skin excision blepharoplasty plus levator aponeurosis repair (resection and/or advancement), and closure without crease creation.

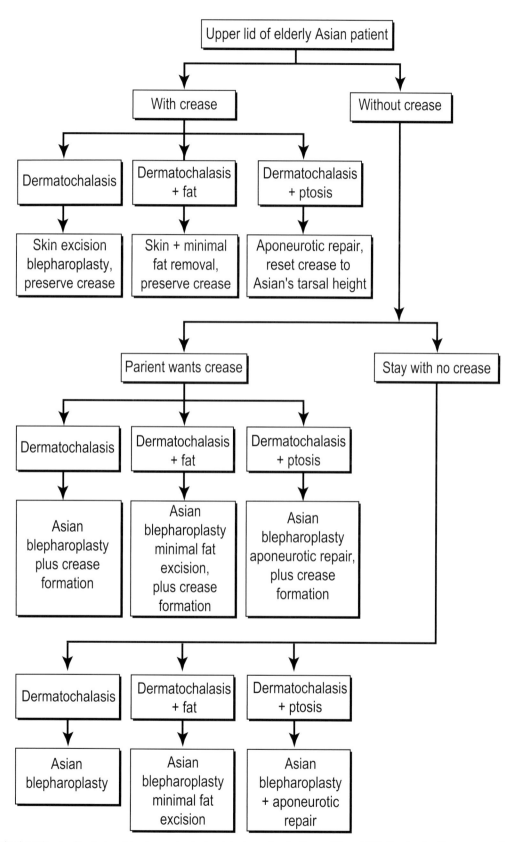

Fig. 8-11 A clinical pathway for Asian blepharoplasty in elderly patients (from Chen WP. Oculoplastic surgery. Stuttgart: Thieme, 2001: 221, Fig.15-18).

Further Reading

1. Chen WPD. Asian blepharoplasty. Ophthalm Plast Reconstruct Surg 1987;3:135–140.
2. Chen WPD. Insights from a series of Asian blepharoplasty. Presented at the Annual Scientific Symposium of the American Society of Ophthalmic Plastic and Reconstructive Surgery, Atlanta, Georgia, 1990.
3. Chen WPD. A comparison of Caucasian and Asian blepharoplasty. Ophthalm Pract 1991;9:216–222.
4. Chen WPD. Upper blepharoplasty in the Asian patient. In: Putterman AM, ed. Cosmetic oculoplastic surgery, 3rd edn. Philadelphia: WB Saunders, 1999: Chapter 11.
5. Chen WPD. Expert commentary on 'Blepharoplasty and blepharoptosis surgery in Asians'. In: Mauriello J, ed. Unfavorable results of eyelid and lacrimal surgery. Oxford: Butterworth–Heinemann, 2000: 68–71.
6. Chen WPD. Concept of triangular, rectangular and trapezoidal debulking of eyelid tissues: application in Asian blepharoplasty. Plast Reconstruct Surg 1996;97:212–218.
7. Chen WPD. Aesthetic eyelid surgery in Asians: an east–west view. Hong Kong J Ophthalmol 2000;3:27–31.
8. Chen WPD (ed). Oculoplastic surgery – the essentials. Stuttgart: Thieme, 2001.
9. Chen WP, Khan J, McCord C. Color atlas of cosmetic oculoplastic surgery. Oxford: Butterworth–Heinemann, 2004.

Advanced Concept of Triangular, Trapezoidal and Rectangular Debulking of Eyelid Tissues – Application in Asian Blepharoplasty

Chapter 9

William P.D. Chen

In previous publications, the author[1-5] discussed the concept of upper eyelid crease configurations and the essential steps required for predictable placement of a lid crease in the eyelids of Asians who do not have a crease. This method is based on accurate measurement of the central height of the upper tarsus, using the measurement to guide the placement of the external incision line for formation of the crease. An aesthetically pleasing crease tends to be either nasally tapered or parallel in configuration. A small medial upper lid fold is often present in the upper eyelids of Asians, whether they have a crease or not, and should not be considered pathologic and automatically removed.

Concept

During Asian blepharoplasty using the external incision method, it is well known that the platform of tissues along the superior tarsal border, if left alone, interferes with the definition and formation of the proposed crease. The various attempts to remove skin,[6] skin with orbicularis muscle,[7,8] skin with pretarsal fat,[9] and skin with muscle and orbital septum and preaponeurotic fat[10,11] all aim to create a clear platform for the formation of adhesions between fibers of the levator aponeurosis and the subcutaneous structure of the surgically produced crease.

Triangular and trapezoidal debulking allows systematic and uniform clearance of the preaponeurotic space along the lower segment of the supratarsal space and its junction with the pretarsal plane. When skin excision (usually measuring less than 2 mm) is performed in conjunction with placement of the lid crease, intraoperative retraction of the upper edge of the skin incision allows an upwardly beveled plane of dissection across the underlying preseptal (supratarsal) orbicularis oculi muscle and the lower portion of the orbital septum. (In Asians who do not have a crease the orbital septum is frequently fused to the levator aponeurosis 2–4 mm above the superior tarsal border; it can be as low as halfway down the anterior surface of the tarsus.) The septum and underlying preaponeurotic fat pads are easily identified.

Trapezoidal Debulking of Preaponeurotic Platform (Fig. 9-1)

The orbital septum is opened horizontally. The trapezoid of preaponeurotic tissues, including an optional and minimal amount of preaponeurotic fat, orbital septum, preseptal orbicularis muscle, subcutaneous fat, and overlying skin (2 mm), all hinging along the superior tarsal border, may be debulked. The anterior surface of this trapezoid is skin only, whereas the posterior portion is wider and includes all preaponeurotic tissues from the septal opening down to the superior tarsal border. A small strand of pretarsal orbicularis muscle along the inferior cut edge of the skin may be trimmed off. Trapezoidal debulking allows easy inward folding of the skin edges towards the underlying aponeurosis for surgical formation of the crease.

There have been scanning electron microscopic studies that described insertions of distal strands of the levator aponeurosis into the subdermal tissue along the lid crease in eyelids that had a crease (see Chapter 3). The formation of a crease is therefore facilitated by the above surgical maneuver, as it links the aponeurosis to the skin overlying the upper edge of the pretarsal platform. Vigorous dissection and debulking of pretarsal tissues is to be avoided, as it tends to lead to persistent edema and the formation of multiple creases.

If debulking is carried out without including any skin excision, the block of tissue removed resembles a triangular configuration in cross-section and may consist of orbicularis and portions of orbital septum.

If the patient has a great deal of skin redundancy the skin included for excision is increased by raising the upper incision line. The plane of dissection through the orbicularis becomes less beveled and more perpendicular, whereas the trapezoidal debulking gradually becomes more of a rectangular configuration.

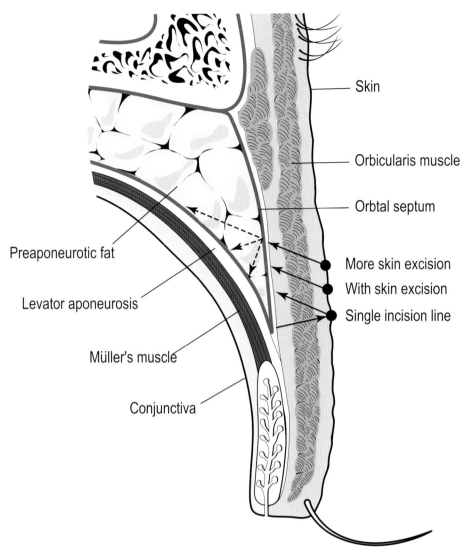

Skin

Orbicularis muscle

Orbtal septum

More skin excision

With skin excision

Single incision line

Preaponeurotic fat

Levator aponeurosis

Müller's muscle

Conjunctiva

Fig. 9-1 Cross-sectional drawing of trapezoidal debulking of the preaponeurotic platform. Black dots correspond to potential lines of skin incision. Solid arrows correspond to transorbicularis vector from skin to orbital septum. Dashed arrows show possible planes of dissection through the preaponeurotic fat pads. Trapezoidal debulking of preaponeurotic tissues in Asian blepharoplasty may include all tissues bounded by the upper (bevelled) and lower (perpendicular) transorbicularis vectors and the tissue between the skin and the orbital septum. Minimal fat excision may be included.

Triangular → Trapezoidal → Rectangular
debulking   debulking   debulking

→ As more skin needs to be removed.

Figure 9-2 (Step 2) shows the bevelled transorbicularis vector for the dissection plane rotating counterclockwise and leveling off as more skin is removed and the upper line of the incision moves further from the superior tarsal border. The shape of the debulked area begins as a triangle and turns into a trapezoid, and finally a rectangle as more skin is removed.

In triangular debulking without skin removal, the ratio (n) of vertical segment of orbicularis to skin removed is many times greater than 1.0 (m ≫ 1).

As debulking proceeds from a trapezoidal to a rectangular configuration, the ratio of vertical segment of orbicularis to skin removed approaches 1:1 (n = 1). The ratio is less than 1.0 only when the amount of redundant skin is quite excessive, as in an elderly person, allowing the removal of excess skin without compromising wound closure or predisposing the patient to ectropion and lagophthalmos of the upper lid. In this situation a 'reverse' trapezoidal block of tissue is removed, the height over the skin side being greater than the height of the preseptal orbicularis muscle excised. Even when a great deal of skin is removed, the traverse through the orbicularis muscle (transorbicularis vector) in an elderly patient should still be perpendicular to the levator palpebrae superioris.

A corollary to this concept is that in young individuals the ratio of orbicularis to skin removed is greater

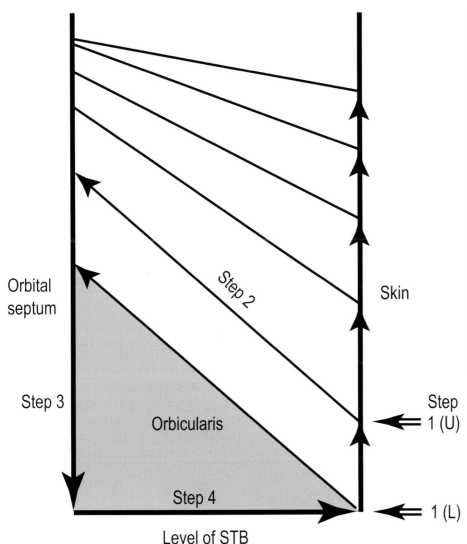

Fig. 9-2 Anterior lamella of upper eyelid; the orbicularis muscle of the supratarsal region and the skin lie anterior to the orbital septum. The first surgical step involves upper and lower lines of incisions [1(U)] and [1(L)] above the superior tarsal border (STB). The second step (2) involves an oblique transection through the orbicularis muscle along the transorbicularis vector line. When the orbital septum is reached and opened in the third step (3), the dissection is carried inferiorly toward the superior tarsal border. Step four (4) is a leveled excision of orbicularis muscle and redundant skin above the superior tarsal border. The transorbicularis vector rotates and levels off as more skin is removed. The cross-section of soft tissues that are debulked changes from triangular to trapezoidal, and finally a rectangular configuration as more skin is removed.

than 1, whereas in elderly individuals it approaches 1:0.

Therefore, in young individuals:

$$\frac{\delta \text{ orbicularis excision}}{\delta \text{ skin excision}} > 1.0$$

In elderly individuals:

$$\frac{\delta \text{ orbicularis excision}}{\delta \text{ skin excision}} = 1.0, \text{ and occasionally } < 1.0$$

Conclusion

The advantages of trapezoidal debulking in Asian blepharoplasty are as follows:

1. Easy approach through the orbital septum when the plane of dissection is beveled. The risk of injury to the levator aponeurosis is reduced when there is a buffer of preaponeurotic fat under the orbital septum.
2. It allows controlled, uniform debulking of the junctional platform between the supratarsal and pretarsal tissues.
3. It allows optimal adhesion between the levator aponeurosis and the inferior subcutaneous tissues, or the intermuscular septa between pretarsal orbicularis muscle fibers (pretarsal platform).
4. It allows crease formation to be based anatomically on the height of the individual tarsus.
5. It reduces the complication rate, including problems related to asymmetry, shape, height,

continuity, permanence, segmentation of the crease due to uneven planes of dissection, fading and late disappearance of the crease, multiple creases, and persistent edema.

References

1. Chen WPD. Asian blepharoplasty. Ophthalmol Plast Reconstruct Surg 1987;3:135–140.
2. Chen WPD. Insights from a series of Asian blepharoplasty. Presented at the Annual Scientific Symposium of the American Society of Ophthalmic Plastic and Reconstructive Surgery, Atlanta, Georgia, 1990.
3. Chen WPD. A comparison of Caucasian and Asian blepharoplasty. Ophthalmol Pract 1991;9:216–222.
4. Chen WPD. Triangular, trapezoidal and rectangular debulking of pre-aponeurotic platform application in Asian blepharoplasty. Plast Reconstruct Surg 1996;97:212–218.
5. Chen WPD, Khan J, McCord CD Jr. Color atlas of cosmetic oculofacial surgery. Oxford: Butterworth–Heinemann, 2004.
6. Sayoe BT. Plastic construction of the superior palpebral fold. Am J Ophthalmol 1954;38:556–559.
7. Hayashi K. The double eyelid operation. Jpn Rev Clin Ophthalmol 1938;33:1000–1010, 1098–1110.
8. Fernandez LR. Double eyelid operation in the oriental in Hawaii. Plast Reconstruct Surg 1960;25:257–264.
9. Inoue S. The double eyelid operation. Jpn Rev Clin Ophthalmol 1947;42:306.
10. Mitsui Y. Plastic construction of a double eyelid. Jpn Rev Clin Ophthalmol 1950;44:19.
11. Sayoc BT. Anatomic considerations in the plastic construction of a palpebral fold in the full upper eyelid. Am J Ophthalmol 1967; 63:155–158.

William P.D. Chen

The various suturing techniques used in external incision methods have already been discussed. They include attaching the skin over the tarsus, attaching the skin towards the levator aponeurosis, along the superior tarsal border, and attaching the inferior orbicularis to the distal portion of the levator aponeurosis.

The Concept of a Dynamic Versus a Static Crease

A dynamic upper lid crease is one that is apparent in straight-ahead gaze and upgaze but which tends to fade on downgaze, and is barely noticeable when viewed at 90° to the skin surface. A static crease would be one that is noticeable in all three positions: upgaze, straight-ahead, and downgaze, when the observing angle is 90°. A dynamic crease therefore resembles a natural crease.

In order to form a dynamic crease, the terminal fibers of the levator aponeurosis above the superior tarsal border must be directed to the subdermal plane of the lower skin incision line. As one is obliged to close the upper skin edge to the lower skin edge, I believe that it is academic to argue on the merits of creating adhesions solely from the terminal aponeurotic fibers to the lower skin edge, or to both the upper and lower skin edges. It is essential to loosen and reposition any adhesive surgical drape that may be used, to allow the upper lid skin to fall along the lower pretarsal skin without tension. The patient is instructed to look up and down to check the adequacy of crease formation and contour before any stitching is begun.

Suturing skin–tarsus–skin tends to yield a static-looking crease. In my technique I use 6/0 non-absorbable silk or nylon interrupted sutures to connect the lower skin edge to the levator aponeurosis along the superior tarsal border, and then to the upper skin edge. Besides the stitch over the center of the crease, I apply three sutures medially and two to three laterally. With these six or seven crease-forming sutures in place,

the rest of the incision may be closed using 6/0 or 7/0 nylon in a continuous or subcuticular fashion. This continuous suture involves only the dermis, without the need to pick up any orbicularis muscle fibers. The objective here would be to avoid hemorrhage from the orbicularis muscle and to provide an optimal plane of closure of the skin incision site. In this method all the sutures are removed.

The method of anchoring inferior subcutaneous tissue alone, or orbicularis to the levator aponeurosis, frequently involves placing buried, non-absorbable sutures. I have come across patients who complain of the static nature of the crease resulting from the use of buried sutures, and some complain of a kinesthetic awareness and often irritation from these buried elements in their eyelids.

Advanced Technique

Crease-Enhancing Maneuvers (McCord's Anchoring/Retention Stitches) (Fig. 8-8)

To enhance or deepen a crease, one may apply three double-armed 5/0 soluble Vicryl sutures transcutaneously from the inferior skin edge to the underlying tarsal plate along the superior tarsal border (applying them over the medial, central and lateral thirds of the eyelid) in addition to regular skin closure. The sutures are then tied externally. After 1 week each of these three knots is trimmed off the skin and the buried loops are left behind. The method works well for non-reactive skin.

Crease Formation and Crease Dynamics

Dynamic Interaction of the Pretarsal Platform and the Preaponeurotic Zone

One can divide the upper eyelid into three zones: the eyelid crease (which acts as the junctional zone or the

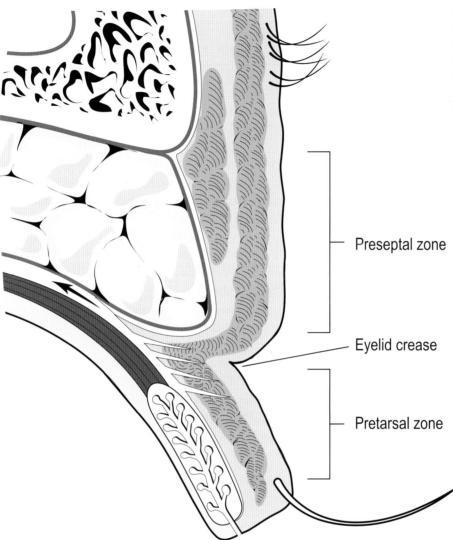

Fig. 10-1 The upper eyelid and crease can be thought of conceptually as consisting of three zones: the eyelid crease (which acts as the junctional zone or the telescoping pivot), the pretarsal zone below it, and the preseptal zone above it.

Preseptal zone

Eyelid crease

Pretarsal zone

telescoping pivot), the pretarsal zone below it, and the preseptal zone above it (Fig. 10-1). The objective of the surgeon in forming or enhancing an upper eyelid crease should be:

1. To facilitate the inward folding of the crease (the pivot) by reducing the soft tissue overlay through limited debulking of redundant preaponeurotic soft tissue, which may be hindering the infolding, or by tightening this pivoting zone through suture ligation (which is less effective by comparison, and more prone to regression). By providing a clear demarcation zone, one achieves a good pivot or telescoping junction.

2. The pretarsal area (lower zone) can be made firmer through (a) excision of some orbicularis oculi muscle along the inferior incisional skin edge, or (b) suture ligation, through conjunctiva to subcutaneous plane buried sutures, or through external skin to levator aponeurosis buried sutures.

3. The fullness of the preseptal area (upper zone) should be preserved by conserving and repositioning most of its preaponeurotic fat superiorly into its sulcus or the upper quadrant of the orbit. There should be no excessive skin removal to avoid foreshortening of the anterior lamella of this upper zone.

These three focal points serve to create an opportunity for the firm pretarsal platform and tarsus (the tarsal–crease unit) to vector upwards and slide under the preseptal soft tissue zone above it, without much effort or encountering any tissue resistance over the crease. The preseptal zone bellows freely over the pretarsal zone, with a crease formed in between.

Conceptually, the crease is thought to form *above* the highest point of insertion of the distal terminations of the levator aponeurosis through the orbicularis oculi's intermuscular septa, as well as skin along the crease line. My trapezoidal debulking approach allows a skin–aponeurosis–skin closure, with a 1–2 mm zone where the transected orbicularis (along the upper beveled skin–muscle wound plane) may become adherent to the aponeurosis just above the superior tarsal border, thereby reforming the 'limiting boundary' previously described as the posterior reflection of the orbital septum's posterior layer on to the levator aponeurosis sheath, and act as an inferior limit to the repositioned preaponeurotic fat. The surgically created crease simply forms directly above this zone. Therefore, although the lid crease wound is formed along the superior tarsal border by taking skin to aponeurosis to skin, the upper lid crease thus formed may lie just above this junction. Another way to conceptualize this is that the aponeurosis is attached to both upper and lower wound skin edges, with the crease thus created lying above it.

Several factors in the upper/preseptal zone can lead to poor infolding of the crease. If fat excision in the preaponeurotic space was excessive, there is now direct physical contact between the aponeurosis and the orbicularis, as the septum has been opened. There is then an attenuation of the preaponeurotic space, which can predispose to cicatrix formation and an increase in rigidity of this zone. If there was inadvertent tissue handling, injury, or above-normal hemorrhaging, there can be increased scarring and consequent rigidity. If there was excessive skin excision in this upper zone, there is a greater probability that the tarsus–eyelid crease unit will be unable to form a crease by telescoping under a structurally tight upper zone. These seemingly benign factors can combine to substantially hinder crease formation.

In Caucasians born with a natural crease, the relatively high point of fusion of the orbital septum on to the levator aponeurosis limits the preaponeurotic fat to above this fusion point. The crease may have formed from either distal terminations of the aponeurosis in towards the inferior orbicularis muscle septa, actual subcutaneous attachment or 'extensions' from the levator, and inferior limitation of fat through a postero-

upward reflection of the posterior layer of the orbital septum on to the levator aponeurosis (this latter scenario may simply yield a prominent supratarsal sulcus in Occidentals who have never had eyelid surgery). This, combined with a softer and thin-skinned preseptal zone, allows the firm tarsal complex to up-vector against it to form a crease.

In Asians with single eyelid, this attempt to form a crease is more difficult for a variety of reasons: the pretarsal soft tissue (skin and boggy orbicularis) is often softer and more redundant; the septum fuses on to the aponeurosis and tarsus at a lower point; preaponeurotic fat is observed concurrently at a lower level; the preseptal zone may have significant fullness and is often positioned more forward in the orbit (Asians have comparatively less deep-set eyes, owing to a less prominent forward extension of the superior orbital rim). These factors are more likely to yield a single lid without a crease.

Following an Asian eyelid crease enhancement procedure, with preservation of fat in the preaponeurotic middle space, coupled with reduction of the pretarsal inferior edge soft tissue, as well as clearance along the superior tarsal border and controlled debulking of the preaponeurotic platform, it will be easier for the crease to fold up. The levator's dynamic pull (up-vector) is most effective when the muscle can glide up against a cushion of non-adherent preaponeurotic fat (middle space) as well as overlying anterior skin–orbicularis. In essence, the tarsal plate and skin are allowed to invaginate against a multilayered soft tissue complex (preaponeurotic fat, septum, orbicularis, subcutaneous fat and skin). It will be more difficult if the preaponeurotic space is obliterated through ablation of its fat, cicatrization between the anterior skin–orbicularis–orbital septum layer and the posterior levator–Müller's muscle–conjunctiva layers through tissue damage or excessive hemorrhage and subsequent hemosiderin deposition. The resultant rigid multilayered tissue complex presents a far greater mass of tissue, as well as a challenge for the tarsal plate to infold against to form a crease. We may see this clinically as a firm band of skin/muscle/anterior lamella in the preseptal region, accompanied by a static-looking crease.

On occasion, postoperative swelling can mask an otherwise well formed crease; and when the swelling resolves the tarsal plate telescopes well against the preseptal soft tissue and a crease then appears appropriately.

The suture ligation methods create a crease by tightening the soft tissue overlying the superior tarsal border, creating a firmer constriction between the subcutaneous skin and the levator aponeurosis (through either an anterior skin or a posterior conjunctival approach). It allows an increased force-gradient where the tarsal plate uplifts in and under the preseptal soft tissues. With no removal of redundant soft tissue, it is effective in the short term (perhaps up to 5 years). However, with aging and a gradual increase in soft tissue redundancy, the crease thus created may become shielded from view or shallow out with time (fading) owing to the unavoidable shredding forces of the buried sutures used in these methods. (The ligatures' effect may diminish in time, not from the dissolution, loosening, or breaking apart of the sutures, but more from the ligature working and cutting through the tissue layers it was meant to tie together.)

A Novel Combined Approach

Partial External Incision Coupled with Buried Orbicularis–Aponeurosis Suture

An ideal procedure and perhaps more time-consuming would be to combine an external incision approach across the central 50% of the proposed area for an eyelid crease, with buried suture ligation over the medial end via the open central wound. This avoids any incision through the thicker medial canthal skin and still achieves a crease as well as control over the shape at the medial extent of the wound, whether the crease is to be nasally tapered or parallel.

Surgical Steps
A corneal protector is applied. The central incision involves excision of a 2–3 mm segment of skin–orbicularis, application of the usual Asian blepharoplasty technique with a beveled approach through the orbicularis and septum, transverse opening of the orbital septum, and minimal excision of preaponeurotic fat, followed by the following.

One may elect to create a subcutaneous tunnel space medially along the superior tarsal border. The location

and hence the height of this medial space will correlate with the desired shape and height of the medial end of the crease. One end of a 6/0 nylon suture is passed through the external skin surface (under magnification using loupes or a microscope) along the desired crease line. It is passed through levator aponeurosis and Müller's muscle, but without penetrating the conjunctiva. It is allowed to travel in a lateral direction for 3 mm, paralleling the crease form. This needle is retrieved through the subcutaneous tunnel space and looped out through the central skin incision wound. One may then choose as follows:

- Option 1: Cut off the second needle of the remaining arm of the suture that has not yet been passed. This end without the needle is then looped through and retrieved within the subcutaneous tunnel space using a strabismus hook. The two ends are tied.
- Option 2: The second needle is left intact and pulled through the skin along the same tract where the first arm passed, and retrieved within the subcutaneous tunnel. It is then rearmed on a needle holder and used to secure small amount of the subcutaneous tissues along the proposed crease line and then tied with the first needle.

Instead of entering the skin through a medial location, a second approach is to come in from a slightly more lateral position but still over the medial third of the uncut eyelid skin. After creating the same subcutaneous tunnel space medially:

- Option 1: The surgeon holds a half-circle needle that is back-armed, and this is passed from a slightly more lateral position through skin and aponeurosis on the bottom of the tunnel space, and then immediately back towards fibers of the subcutaneous tissues over the top of the tunnel space to form a complete 270° loop. This contains the tissues along the superior tarsal border as well as subcutaneous tissues. The second arm is pulled through the skin without its needle, and the two suture ends are tied and buried.
- Option 2: The back-armed needle approaches the skin and levator aponeurosis laterally. It is retrieved within the subcutaneous tunnel space, rearmed, and used to secure some subcutaneous fascial tissues on the top of the tunnel space. The

second arm is pulled through without its needle, and the two ends are tied and buried.

The passage of needle through a tight and vascular compartment will lead to occasional hemorrhage from the orbicularis and is certainly a factor in terms of assessing the efficacy of the procedure.

The location of the medial end of the crease thus created depends on where the subcutaneous tunnel is fashioned and where the buried stitches are applied. For a nasally tapered crease that converges normally, the medial end of the crease is usually applied at distance from the lid margin equal to two-thirds of the measured central height of the tarsal plate. When there is a coincidental medial canthal fold this maneuver will uplift the medial lid fold. For those patients who desire a rapidly converging nasally tapered crease (rapidly tapering), one may place the medial end of the crease at one-third of the measured central height of the tarsus. This is lower than the actual height of the tarsal plate there, though the needle should still be aimed towards aponeurotic fibers along the medial aspect of the superior tarsal border.

Over the central skin incision, which spans 50% of the normal crease, the wound is closed using four interrupted 6/0 silk sutures in the usual fashion for Asian blepharoplasty, taking lower skin–aponeurosis–upper skin. There will be four external stitches over an area of about 13–14 mm. The lateral quarter of the eyelid skin is uncut and has no buried sutures. The medial end is also uncut, but has a buried suture to help form the medial end of the crease without any risk of residual hypertrophic scarring.

A further option relates to the placement of the central skin incision. One can maintain a 50% width incision but shift it laterally, such that the medial end of the eyelid has an uncut skin zone of about 10 mm, rather than 7 mm as above. This has the added advantage of allowing a greater resection of the lateral orbicularis and skin, as there is often a greater level of hooding and redundancy there. These excess tissues need to be debulked to avoid subsequent fading of the crease laterally.

The essentials for this combined approach are:

1. The whole length of the crease should be marked (centrally this becomes the lower skin incision line). This helps in coordinating the central crease with the medial crease to avoid truncation of the crease. The use of a corneal protector is mandatory.
2. The buried medial suture should be applied under magnification and direct vision. Be mindful of the superior tarsal arcade as well as Müller's blood vessels.
3. There is little preaponeurotic fat medially that may potentially interfere with crease formation.
4. The levator is relatively ineffective in the medial one-quarter zone. It is more fibrous in nature, and converges with the pretarsal and preseptal orbicularis to form the medial canthal ligamentous complex.
5. A lateral shift of this limited skin incision allows excision of skin laterally.
6. Buried medial sutures avoid incision scars through the thick medial canthal skin.
7. The medial canthal buried suture approach can always be converted or approached later on through an open incisional approach, should the need arise.

The levator located over the central one-third of the upper eyelid has good dynamic excursion and is measurable as levator function in a normal individual. It is apparent that the vertical excursion of the levator is maximal over the central area of the upper eyelid, and this is why some small central incision methods with partial excision of fat also seem to work. The medial third of the width of the eyelid has fibers of levator aponeurosis, but this has relatively little vertical movement. A surgically applied crease here will need to rely on passive fixation of skin to the underlying aponeurosis, or fixation of the orbicularis to the levator aponeurosis. The lateral one-third of the levator aponeurosis likewise has very little vertical excursion, and mostly coalesces with the lateral extent of the pretarsal and preseptal orbicularis muscle to form the fibrous lateral canthal raphe. Crease formation here often depends on skin–orbicularis fixation.

There are further surgical options involving these non-incisional methods of crease formation that require delivery through an open skin incision centrally:

1. Within the medial subcutaneous tunnel space created via a central skin incision, one may apply bipolar cautery with tying forceps tips to cauterize

the epitarsal tissues (from midtarsal height to the upper superior tarsal border) to create a tightened platform.

2. Excision of subcutaneous soft tissues can be carried out medially using an Ellemann radiofrequency unit (with Empire needle tip) for precise tissue excision, or monopolar cautery with Colorado needle tip. Bipolar cautery can be added to supplement hemostatic control.

3. Excision of subcutaneous soft tissues can be similarly carried out laterally within a subcutaneous tunnel space, again created via a central skin incision using an Ellemann radiofrequency unit with Empire needle tip for precise tissue excision, or monopolar cautery with Colorado needle tip. Here in the lateral quadrant, buried orbicularis–aponeurotic sutures may be used, bearing in mind the abundance of orbicularis fibers and the vascularity here.

Kim and Lee[1] have described the use of Nd-YAG laser in dealing with the medial and lateral ends of their Asian blepharoplasty cases.

Figures 10-2 to 10-13 are preoperative and postoperative photos illustrating cases of typical Asian Blepharoplasty surgery with expected outcomes.

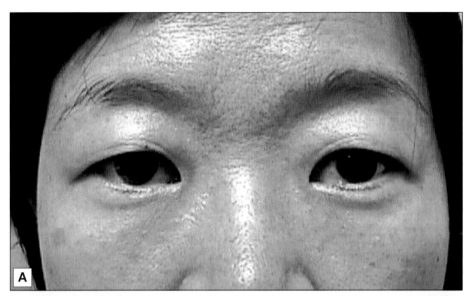

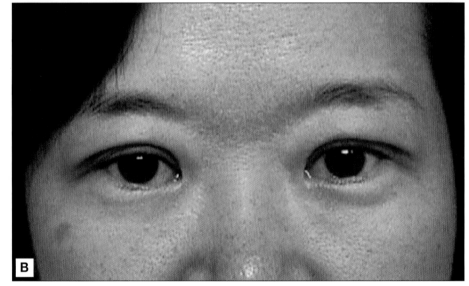

Fig. 10-2

Fig. 10-3

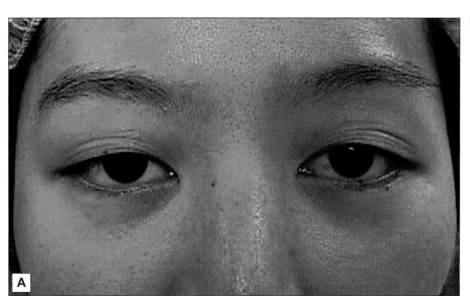

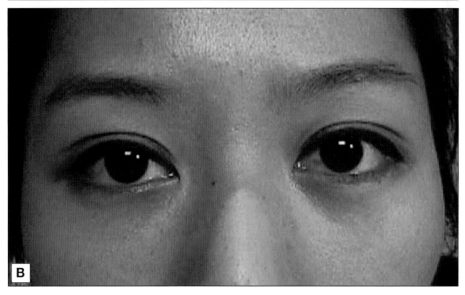

Fig. 10-4

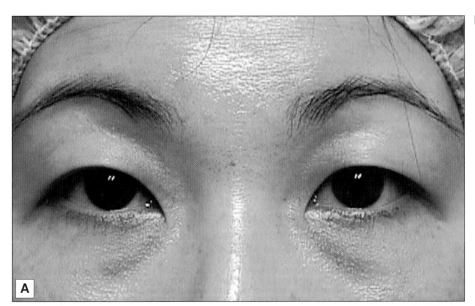

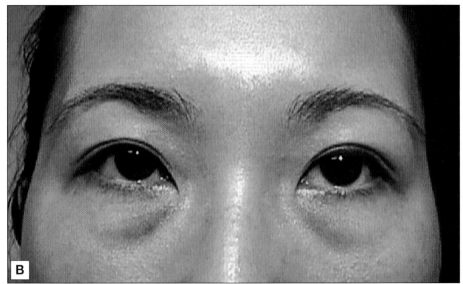

Fig. 10-5

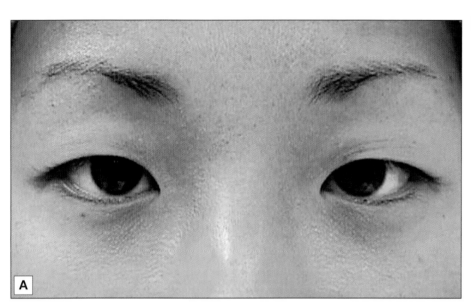

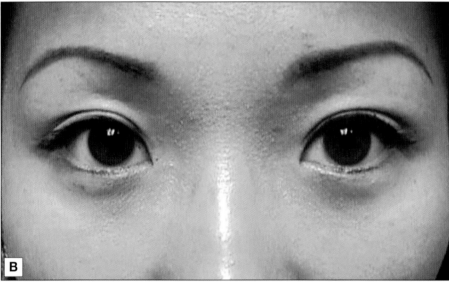

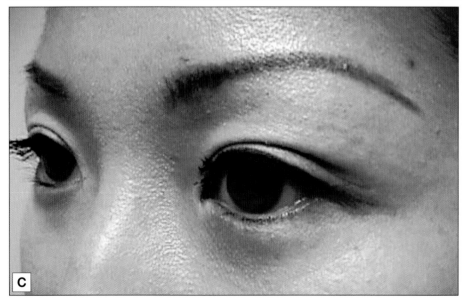

Fig. 10-6

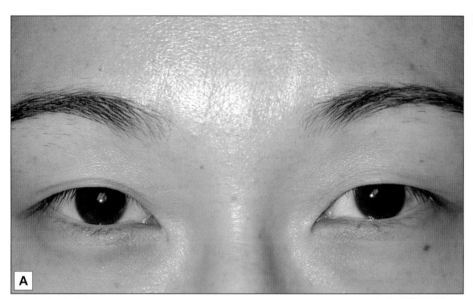

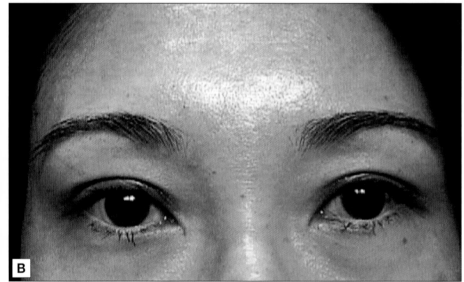

Fig. 10-7

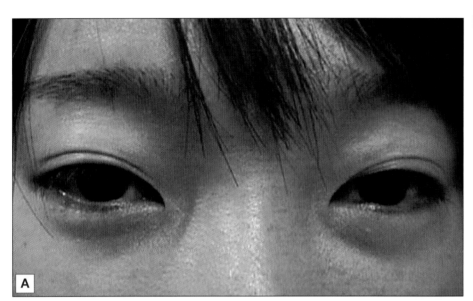

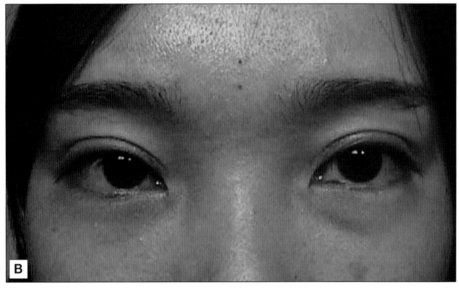

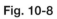
Fig. 10-8

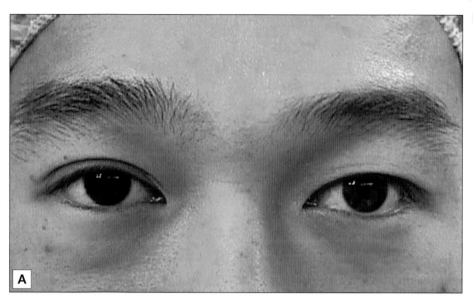

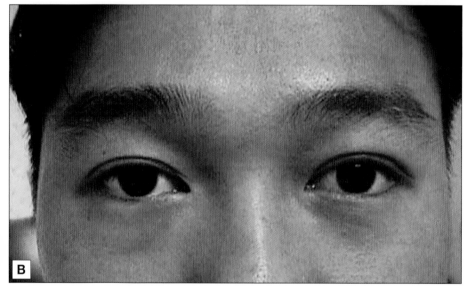

Fig. 10-9

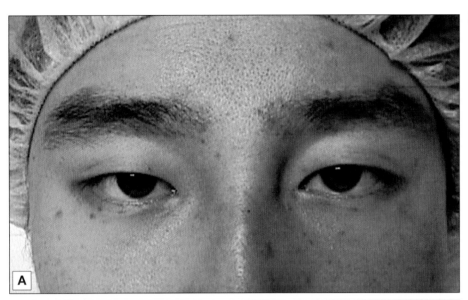

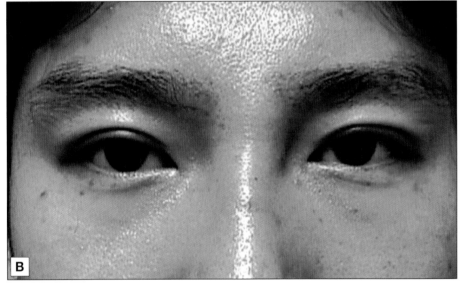

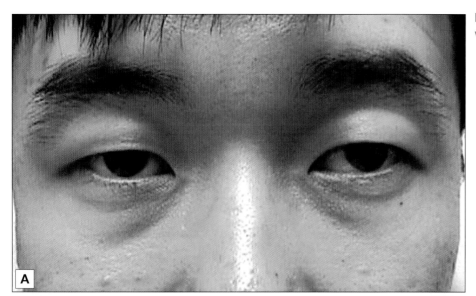

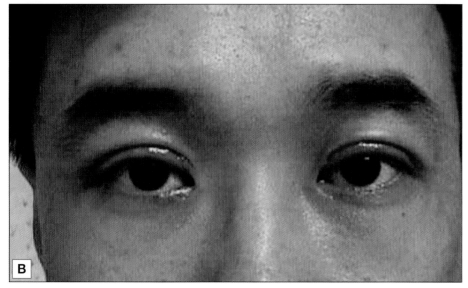

Fig. 10-10 Before and after view at one week postoperative visit.

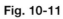

Fig. 10-11

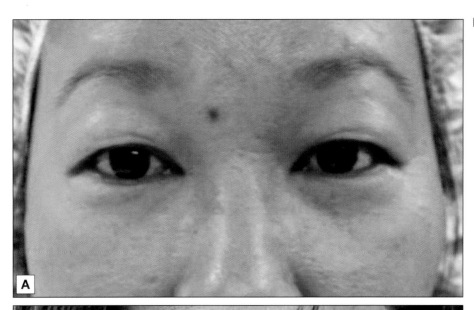

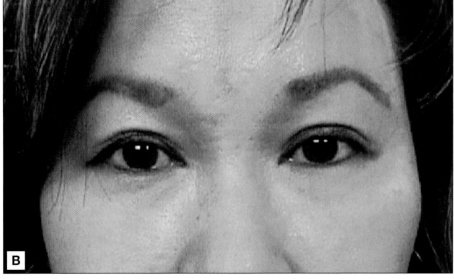

Fig. 10-12

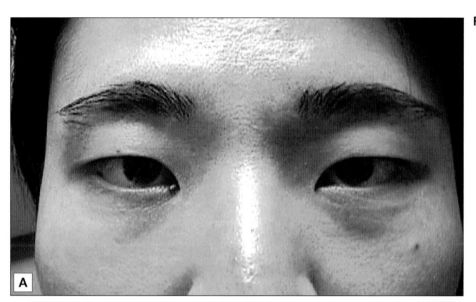

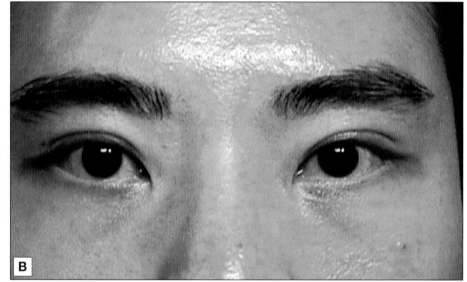

Fig. 10-13

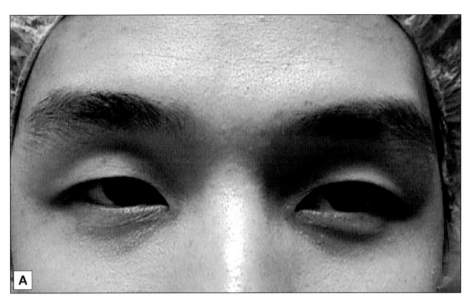

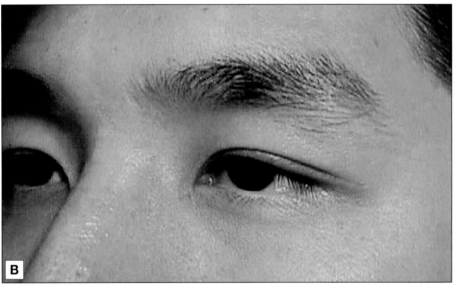

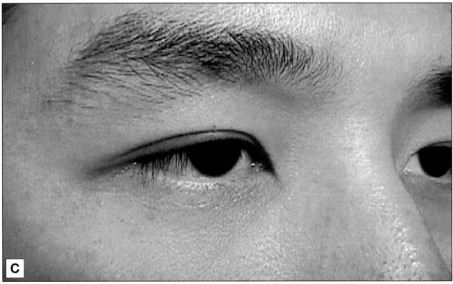

Reference

Kim JW, Lee JO. Asian blepharoplasty with a short-pulsed contact Nd-YAG laser: limited-incision resectable laser double fold with internal medial and lateral functional epicanthoplasty. Aesthetic Plast Surg 1998;22:433–438.

Postoperative Care

Chapter 11

William P.D. Chen

During the immediate postoperative period the wound is cleaned daily and covered with antibiotic ointment. Compressive or occlusive eye dressings are to be avoided. Diuretics and steroids are not usually prescribed. Depending on the material used, the sutures are removed 5–7 days after the operation. I may leave in interrupted sutures (skin–levator aponeurosis–skin) for a slightly longer period if the crease seems slow in forming, as this seems to help ensure proper attachment of the levator aponeurosis to the incision line along the superior tarsal border.

About 80% of the postoperative swelling should have disappeared a week after the sutures are removed, or at 2 weeks postoperatively. The remaining 20% will regress by 2 months. The crease migrates closer to the ciliary margin when pretarsal tissue edema subsides as a result of lymphatic and vascular rechanneling. Patients are told that even if all goes well their surgically placed crease will take 3–6 months to stabilize.

Should there be a need for revision touch-up, for example if the crease does not form distinctively, the author performs this no earlier than 6 months, as the crease continues to mature. The author does not advocate secondary revision in patients seeking consultation after having had previous procedure(s) elsewhere unless a 12-month period has elapsed.

The patient is given a short list of instructions to follow postoperatively.

Postoperative Regimen for Asian Blepharoplasty Patients

- Bed rest for 24 hours
- Ice compresses for 1 day
- No reading, watching of television or computer use. No computer-gaming
- Wound and facial hygiene: clean face and incision wounds three to four times daily with clean water
- Avoid the use of cosmetics over the incision wound and sutures
- Apply antibiotic ointment four times daily for 7 days
- Patient may shower that day
- Avoid hot-spa or swimming
- Avoid strenuous activities or workout for at least 1 week
- Avoid aspirin compounds or anything containing ibuprofen
- Avoid spicy food, chocolate, dairy products and fried foods for 2 months.

Crease-Enhancing Eye Exercises for Patients without a Pre-Existing Crease

Practice excursion of the upper lids, from downgaze to upgaze, without involving the brow and forehead muscles and without allowing the head to be tilted backwards in any way, starting on the third day after the operation and continuing for 2 weeks. These exercises help initiate formation of the lid crease in selected patients. The levator movement should be deliberately slow in order to allow good crease infolding without pulling on any fine blood vessels and causing postoperative hematoma.

The last point bears further explanation: some patients may have such low pain tolerance that they dare not look up or even straight ahead, as the skin sutures may cause some local irritation. They may be in a head-tilted-back position all week without activating any levator movement or upgaze. The crease may not form well if there have been no attempts at upgaze during the first 10 days. This form of eye movement is best performed slowly, hence the term 'Eye-Chi' coined by the author (as in the slow graceful excursions of Tai-Chi). It is important to initiate upgaze and thereby contract the levator muscle to assist in forming a proper crease. Slow daily movement of the eyelids helps reduce the swelling over the pretarsal and preseptal regions. It also helps ingrain muscle memory, as a number of patients who lack a crease also have a relative inability for full upgaze, and a still smaller percentage

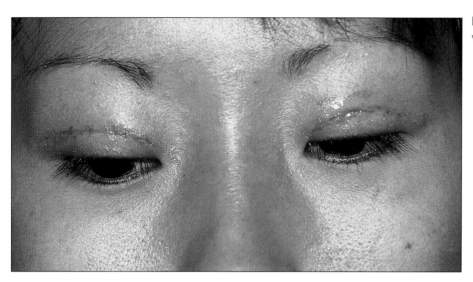

Fig. 11-1 Natural wound induration visible 1 week postoperatively.

may have a concomitant ptosis, although this is usually mild and often subclinical, their levator function often being less than 10 mm. Such muscle memory training may be entirely new for these patients. It helps them become aware that they often have an overaction of their forehead and eyebrows to start with.

The surgeon should expect panic calls from patients and should provide reassurance. I often see my patients more frequently than is medically necessary to help allay their concerns.

The importance of meticulous attention to the contour and placement of the crease cannot be overemphasized. These factors are dictated by the design of the incision line and the placement of the interrupted sutures on the levator aponeurosis. One must diligently avoid the construction of an excessively high crease, or one that is too deep or too harsh. One might avoid the removal of an excessive amount of preaponeurotic fat. I also avoid excising any supracanthal web of skin (medial upper lid fold).

When the sutures are removed, whether all at once or in two separate stages several days apart, it is not unusual to see tissue induration over the incision wound and the suture tracts (Fig. 11-1). Partly because the sutures that anchor the lid crease are under tension, the dermal reaction may be more intense than one would normally expect. When I encounter this type of reaction I prescribe a short course of topical fluometholone (FML) ophthalmic ointment to be applied over the crease incision. These indurations tend to regress within several weeks; reactions such as

hypertrophic scarring tend to linger much longer. According to the literature, keloids are seldom seen over the upper eyelids. I have found this to be true, having seen no true keloid formation over the crease. The same is not true of keloid formation over the thicker skin of the medial canthal region, however, where very prominent scars from attempts at medial canthoplasty, intercanthal fixation, and even VY-plasty have been observed.

Patients may still present with a variety of concerns or complaints, which may include:

1. Unevenness of the crease, even within the first hours, day or week. This is often caused by different degrees of swelling between the two lids. It may be in the pretarsal area, which will broaden a crease, or in the preseptal and periorbital region, which may depress and diminish the apparent width of a crease. Often postoperatively the width of the crease may be influenced by the position of the side of the face during sleep: the dependent side will tend to have correspondingly more edema and therefore the crease may appear broader, owing to pretarsal fullness.

2. A crease may not appear to be adequately folded in after sutures were removed at 1 week postoperatively. The explanation could be residual swelling, or newly formed swelling can temporarily shallow out a crease.

3. A crease may still appear to be hooded or shielded even after surgery: this is likely to be due to

preseptal tissue swelling overhanging the crease.

4. Bleeding and hematoma beyond the first 2 days. This happens infrequently, but usually arises from excessive physical activities several days after surgery.

5. Infection, cellulitis, erysipelas, accompanied by redness, itching, and tenderness to touch.

6. Itching, usually due to allergic dermatitis or a reaction to topical antibiotic ointment.

7. Crease not folding in well over the medial one-third of the lid margin: the skin–levator attachment may be suboptimal, the levator muscle may not be well formed medially, or the swelling may have temporarily obliterated the infolding of the crease. The crease may still appear after 2–3 months.

8. Late complaints:
   - Induration over the medial one-third of the incision wound (the dermis is thicker there)
   - Suture tract cyst formation
   - Blackhead (comedo) formation from early use of cosmetics during the postoperative period
   - Wound dehiscence (rare)
   - Persistent fullness over the pretarsal area (rare if the Asian blepharoplasty techniques mentioned in this text are followed)
   - Chemosis of conjunctiva (rare).

In general, the postoperative care of Asian patients who undergo cosmetic upper lid operations requires patience and understanding on the part of both patient and surgeon. Patients should understand the normal healing course for Asian eyelid skin, so that they have a proper time frame in which to observe the progression of wound healing. Surgeons should be understanding of the patient's psychological needs and of their anxiety, should provide ample reassurance, and should render sound medical care in the extended postoperative period.

Suboptimal Results and Parameters of Complications

William P.D. Chen

Chapter 12

The revision of suboptimal results is a necessary part of any surgeon's skills. Known factors that lead to suboptimal results include inaccurate placement of the crease incision, the use of reactive suture materials, excessive bleeding, excessive fat removal, inadequate or excessively tight wound closure, inappropriate technique, and lack of knowledge on the part of the surgeon.

There are often intangible factors that may be beyond the control of the surgeon. Examples are the patient's lack of compliance with postoperative wound care instructions; overly vigorous physical exercises performed too soon after the procedure, resulting in prolonged edema of the eyelid margin; latent hypertension with rebleeding; weight gain; unpredictable wound healing in patients who have had multiple prior revisions; obsession on the part of patients who are not happy with the results even though the results are satisfactory; or unrealistic preconceived notions on the part of patients about what they expect the crease to do for them, such as launching a career in a certain field.

Assuming the physician is knowledgeable and capable, deviations from an ideal course may still occur inadvertently or even unnoticed, arising from an unusual pairing of an event from the patient and an event from the physician. Suboptimal results may therefore occur even with the very best surgeon.

A physician may not be aware that his patient has anemia, or a low platelet count, or poor coagulative function, was on aspirin therapy, or was consuming herbal remedies. During surgery, intraoperative bleeding may thus be significant and disruptive. This requires extra countermeasures using unipolar or bipolar cautery. Under local anesthesia that same patient may become even more anxious and the blood pressure may escalate, resulting in the formation of a hematoma. Cautery and aggressive manipulation to reach the source of the bleeding blood vessel often results in postoperative ptosis. This further compromises the ability of the eyelid to form the desired crease. Swelling of tissue planes can result in unevenness of the crease, resembling the segmentation seen in bamboo, or crease asymmetry between the two sides. It may even cause an incision line to appear crooked, even though the surgeon has perfectly stable hands. An overly anxious patient may suddenly become claustrophobic and move during a critical part of the incision or excision process, resulting in a less than ideal outcome. The Asian blepharoplasty procedure requires total concentration, and even a friendly and talkative patient or innocent questions from staff in the operating theater may distract the surgeon.

There are other scenarios when physicians have absolutely nothing to do with the untoward outcome of particular cases, for example:

- A slender young woman underwent successful Asian blepharoplasty. She was happy and apparently gained 30lb upon recovery from her borderline anorexia nervosa, and the crease on one side of the eye became obliterated. This required an enhancement procedure, with further excision of her newly gained preseptal fat pads.

- A dentist had undergone successful Asian blepharoplasty. Six months postoperatively he went camping in the wilderness for a week and was bitten by an unknown insect over the lid margin. That upper lid crease became shallow and the pretarsal tissues broadened, resulting in a higher crease on that same eyelid. It required a revision to reset the crease to a lower level.

- A 30-year-old lawyer developed erysipelas during the latter half of the first week after surgery. Both creases turned red and the pretarsal segment became wider, accompanied by scaly eruptions over the cheek skin area. A systemic oral antibiotic was used and the infection promptly subsided.

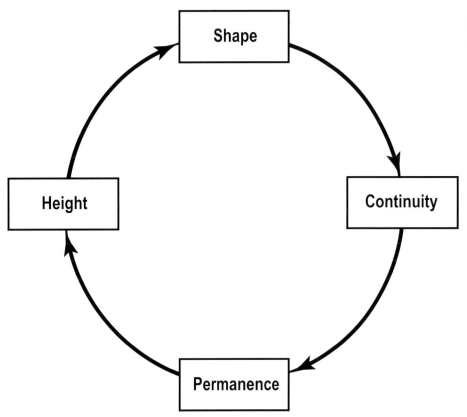

Fig. 12-1 Interrelated parameters that determine a normal crease as well as suboptimal results.

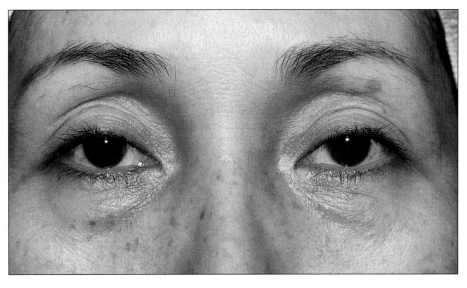

Fig. 12-2 Hollow sulcus as a result of excessive removal of preaponeurotic fat.

An Undesirable Crease

An undesirable crease can be analyzed in a logical manner. The four factors that determine a crease are also the ones that may lead to a suboptimal crease: height, shape, continuity, and permanence (Fig. 12-1).

Height

The crease may be placed too high or too low, each presenting unique problems. A high crease is often seen in conjunction with overzealous removal of preaponeurotic fat pads. It results in a high supratarsal sulcus or a 'famined' look that is difficult to correct (Fig. 12-2). For a patient who has a slight hollow below the

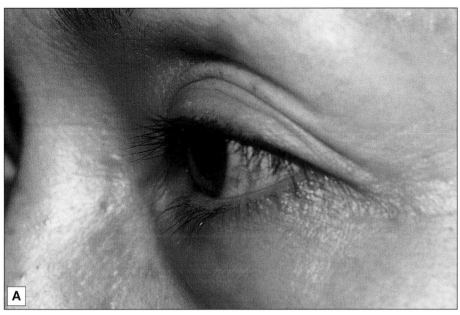

Fig. 12-3 (A, B) Formation of multiple creases and false folds as a result of excessive fat removal.

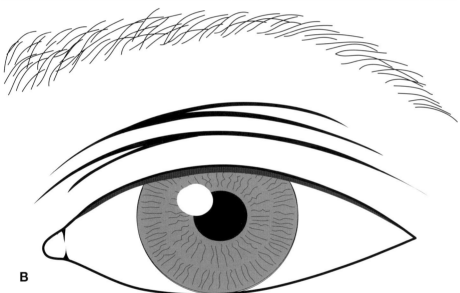

superior orbital rim preoperatively, the removal of preaponeurotic fat may give rise to a prominent supratarsal sulcus and the formation of multiple skin folds over the high crease (Fig. 12-3A, B). In this situation the removal of more skin to eliminate these folds without addressing the problem of the sulcus usually leads to an even greater degree of deformity.

Shape

The problems related to shape are discussed in Chapter 3. The face may appear incongruous if a semilunar (half-moon) crease is applied to an Asian eyelid

(Fig. 12-4). In operations to produce a nasally tapered crease in the eyes of patients who have a small medial canthal web (medial upper lid fold), if the medial extent of the crease was not deliberately tailored to merge under the web and has come to be located above it, the result may be an upper bifid crease over the medial end of the crease (Fig. 12-5). If the medial portion of the crease is overly tapered and has come to be located inferior to the medial canthal web, a rare lower bifid crease is seen. The author has seen patients in whom the lateral portion of a crease was flared up excessively from the lateral canthus, encroaching on the thicker dermis of the eyebrow area.

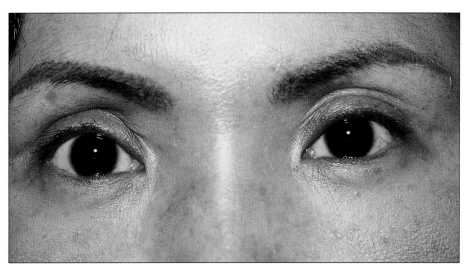

Fig. 12-4 Excessively high semilunar crease.

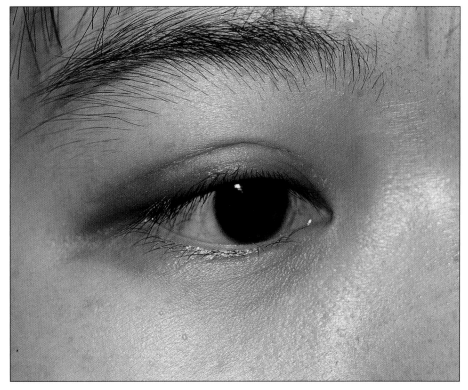

Fig. 12-5 Upper bifid crease 1 month postoperatively. With time and resolution of tissue edema the bifid crease may merge into the medial upper lid fold.

Continuity and Permanence

Problems associated with continuity are linked to permanence in the following way. If the crease is not well connected to its underlying aponeurosis in a continuous manner, it may present as a discontinuous or broken crease and become evident soon after the operation. A continuous crease may be well formed initially but then became obliterated, resulting in a shallow crease or no crease at all – in essence a nonpermanent crease; or the crease may break apart later in a segmental manner, becoming discontinuous

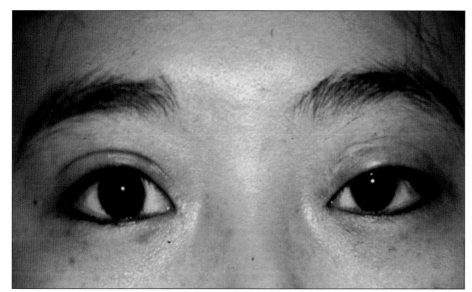

Fig. 12-6 Lid crease placement by the external incision method. The right upper crease covers about 80% of the width of the lid. The left lid crease has become obliterated.

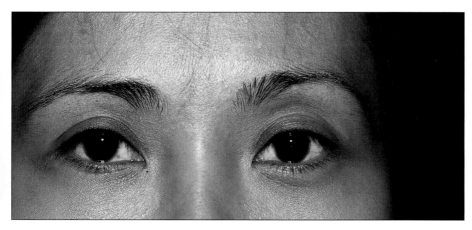

Fig. 12-7 Postoperative formation of multiple creases over the pretarsal region of the left upper lid. The most likely cause of this suboptimal result is vigorous surgical maneuvering in the pretarsal region.

but permanent (Fig. 12-6). The incidence of crease disappearance appears to be much higher when the suture ligation methods are used.

Patients who have multiple creases often have had more than one operation. The multiple creases arise from unpredictable scar formation after reoperations, and from an excessive degree of dissection in the pretarsal region of the upper eyelid (Fig. 12-7).

Finally, I have worked with several patients who desired to have their surgically placed creases reversed.

Circle of Complications and Parameters, Etiology and Interrelatedness

Of all the parameters that influence the outcome of surgery, perhaps the single most important factor that draws attention will be the height of the crease, as drawn from the mid-ciliary margin. The crease should be designed based on the central height of the tarsal plate, and no higher. In Asians this is often between 6.5 and 8.0 mm. When designed in this range the crease often proves natural in appearance and well formed. When designed above the measured height of the tarsus, the result is often a crease that is unnatural in appearance, restrictive in upgaze, and associated with increased lymphedema in the pretarsal region, manifesting as a 'fat' eyelid border. A crease that is designed lower than the lowest range of normal will often lead to a scar in the pretarsal skin region which is hard to camouflage, or the lymphatic stasis and eventual resolution lead to multiple creases and folds (Fig. 12-8).

Next in importance is the shape of the crease design, i.e. nasally tapered or parallel. The nasally tapered crease is popular and compatible with almost any Asian ethnicity. Its distinctive feature is a gradual convergence towards the medial canthus, and it may simply converge without joining or may join the medial canthal angle. As it courses medially, the indented crease would join and merge towards any mild medial canthal fold the patient may already have. The nasally tapered crease seems more prevalent in southern Chinese, as well as in southeastern ethnic groups such as Malaysians, Thais, Vietnamese, and Cambodians. The parallel crease is more often seen in northern Chinese as well as northern Asians. The crease is uniform in width as it arches from one corner of the lid to the other. It appears to be aesthetically more compatible for someone with larger facial features, a more rectangular or squarish face, or someone who is tall and hence has a proportionately larger face. The parallel crease may be observed among southern Asians and the nasally tapered crease may likewise be seen in northerners. If a crease is designed with the correct shape but with a height above the normal range, it becomes conspicuous and artificial in appearance. When a crease is designed without following the nor-mal geometric contour for that particular crease shape, again one has the impression of artificiality, for example a crease that flares up medially, or one that converges laterally (both opposite to what may normally occur in those locations). This applies when one is comparing the symmetry of design between two eyelids: again it would be less than ideal to have a crease shape on one side that differs from what is on the opposite side (although this is far less suboptimal in the overall scheme). There are times when a surgeon finds that a semicircular crease is created unintentionally on one side and the desired crease on the other. This can be revised back to the desired shape at the appropriate time, provided there are some skin reserves to work with.

During the design as well as the construction phase of the crease, and especially for a nasally tapered crease, if the surgeon does not steer the medial end towards and merge with the medial canthal fold a bifid crease can be the result – a crease that splits either above or below the medial canthal fold.

An artificially high crease incision will naturally lead one to encounter a greater amount of fat in the preaponeurotic space because of its high entry. There is a chance that the surgeon will then be unknowingly steered towards a greater than normal degree of fat excision. This leads to:

1. A more hollowed preseptal region (enhanced supratarsal sulcus);
2. A greater chance of the formation of multiple creases or folds above the lower incision line, in the preseptal region. There is then a confusing picture of competing creases, rather than a predominant and primary crease being formed;
3. A greater chance of a comparatively rigid preseptal segment of skin–muscle–posterior lamella.

It is therefore apparent that excess fat excision has a multiplying and cascading effect in terms of its influence on eventual formation of the lid crease. Not only does it not help in crease formation or the eventual aesthetics of the upper eyelid, it makes subsequent revision attempts far more challenging.

Continuity relates to factors in the construction of a crease: the efforts must be uniform and deliberate, with varying techniques tailored to the particular terrain across the width of the eyelid fissure. If the effort

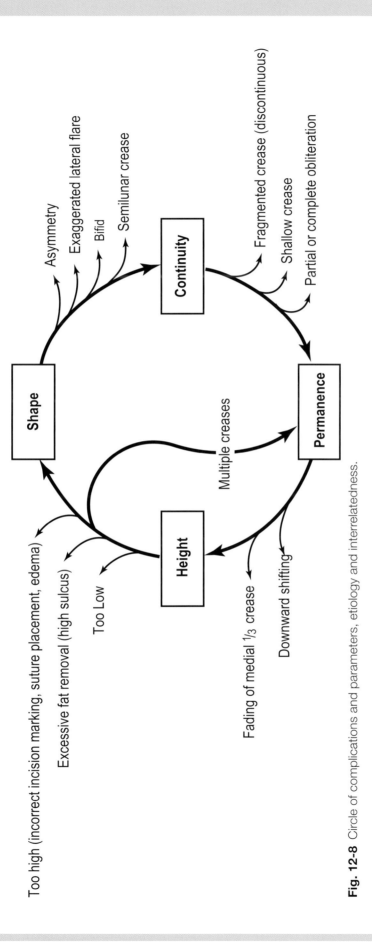

Fig. 12-8 Circle of complications and parameters, etiology and interrelatedness.

should succeed in most of the length of the crease but fail in a small location, the result is a discontinuous or partial crease (or a partially obliterated crease). The crease may become indistinct, either medially, centrally (less often), or laterally.

Permanence refers to the ideal goal of achieving a crease that remains for more than 3–5 years. When the entire crease fades out over a 6-month period it is usually due to insufficient clearance of the soft tissue corridor along the preaponeurotic platform, with regression of the soft tissue barrier, including fat, along the zone where the crease would ideally form. It can also occur as a result of an excessively low incision path along the pretarsal plane.

Continuity, therefore, relates more to the overall effort of crease fixation, assuming the path is already on the correct level and plane. Permanence includes the effort made to ensure continuity but relates to long-term success and the efficacy of a particular method, as applied to an individual patient.

The challenge is that with any of the factors mentioned above and shown in the circle of factors, each one may have a slight imperfection that can lead to less than perfect results. Aggregation of several suboptimal factors can pose a greater degree of challenge when it comes to revision attempts. It is not uncommon to see revision attempts at the excision of multiple folds or a high crease lead to severe skin shortage, lagophthalmos, and corneal exposure. Likewise, injection of free fat grafts may lead to mechanical ptosis, hypertrophy of injected fat, or lumpy fat grafts. Acquired ptosis is a common sequela following revision attempts and can be cicatricial (owing to high crease fixation) or mechanical (stiffened preseptal platform) in origin. Scarring in the middle lamella and involving the levator muscle can lead to both lagophthalmos and ptosis, as well as poor closure of the palpebral fissure and corneal exposure.

Revision and Correction of Suboptimal Results – Advanced Concepts

Chapter 13

William P.D. Chen

It is hoped that with knowledge, skill, and careful pre-operative discussion, the surgeon can avoid the factors that lead to suboptimal results. This chapter will discuss some of the problems the author has encountered in the treatment of patients who seek revisions, and their solutions.

Revision Techniques

The revision techniques for the various suboptimal configurations are discussed below.

Crease Asymmetry

By far the most frequently encountered problem is crease asymmetry. This includes creases that are unequal in height (Fig. 13-1), uneven in shape and continuity, have undergone shifting (downward migration or partial or complete obliteration of the crease) (see Fig. 13-6), or have faded in the medial one-third of the lid (Fig. 13-2).

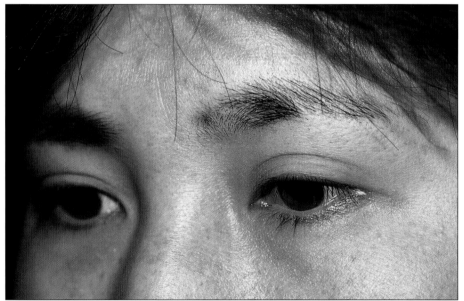

Fig. 13-1 Asymmetric creases (left crease higher than right).

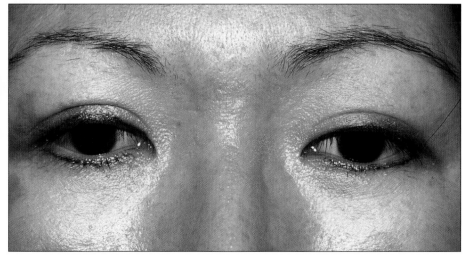

Fig. 13-2 Fading of medial third of left upper lid crease.

Inequality in Crease Height

When the crease of one eyelid appears higher than that of the other, often the higher crease is the abnormal one. It is essential to detect any acquired ptosis in that eyelid, because the levator aponeurosis often appears to have dehisced some of its lower terminal interdigitations and has only a portion of its superior lid crease attachments remaining (Fig. 13-3). Correction of the ptosis eliminates the apparently higher crease without any need to reposition the crease.

A higher than normal crease can arise from inappropriate marking of the incision lines, from inaccurate placement of the interrupted crease-forming sutures over the levator aponeurosis, or from persistent edema in the pretarsal plane. If a crease still appears high 6–9 months after the operation, the repair can be accomplished in the following manner.

Repair of a High Crease

The eyelid is everted and the central height of the tarsus measured (see Chapter 7). This serves as a reference point for crease placement. When the tarsal height is transposed on the skin side and is found to be closer to the eyelash line than the current crease, the difference in millimeters of skin can be excised with the previous incision scar, as long as a shortage of skin does not result and complete eyelid closure is not compromised (Fig. 13-4). It is helpful to lyze any subcutaneous aponeurotic attachment along the superior edge of the incision. Any scar tissue that may overlie the aponeurotic attachment along the superior tarsal border should be removed to allow for the construction of the new crease.

If the transcribed tarsal height on the skin side is higher than the supposedly high crease, one should examine the contralateral upper lid crease to see if it has an excessively low crease.

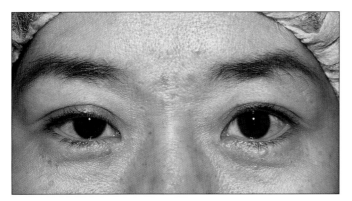

Fig. 13-3 Acquired ptosis of the right upper eyelid and a higher crease compared to the left upper lid. The crease asymmetry is corrected when the underlying ptosis is corrected.

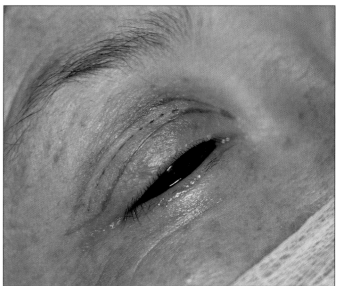

Fig. 13-4 This patient had a higher than acceptable crease (dotted line); it was corrected by Asian blepharoplasty.

Low Crease

It is more difficult to repair an excessively low crease (one that is close to the lash margin) than to repair an excessively high one. The correction is tailored to whether there is any redundancy of skin.

Repair of a Low Crease

For patients who have some redundant skin, the best method is simple excision of the scar associated with the low crease, allowing it to heal, and then performing a subsequent crease procedure a minimum of 6 months later. In my experience, simultaneous revision and construction of a new crease often gives suboptimal control of crease height.

When the skin is taut and has no redundancy, simple excision cannot be performed because it may result in cicatricial ectropion or a prominent scar (Fig. 13-5). An acceptable option for a low crease with a scarcity of skin is complete excision of the crease and the adjacent pretarsal skin, replacing them with a full-thickness skin graft and reshaping the crease at the same time. This procedure is used if the graft covers only the pretarsal region. The patient should be forewarned that the crease will appear high for at least 6 months.

If the skin graft required spans both the pretarsal and the supratarsal regions, it is best to defer crease reconstruction for at least 6 months (Fig. 13-6).

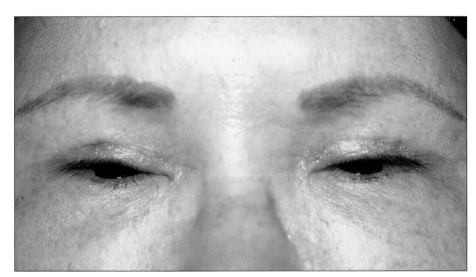

Fig. 13-5 Mild cicatricial retraction and prominent scar.

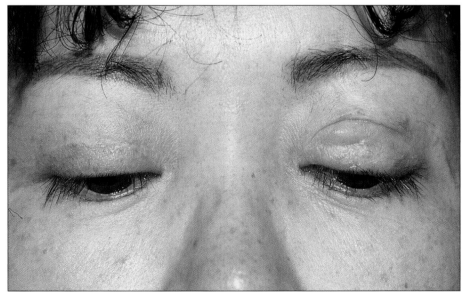

Fig. 13-6 Cicatricial retraction and corneal exposure that necessitated skin grafting superior to the pretarsal region. Plan for the formation of a lid crease is deferred for at least 6 months.

Late Obliteration of a Crease

Late obliteration includes a shallow crease, shifting of a crease, fading of the medial third of a crease, and obliteration of the entire crease (Fig. 13-7).

Repair of Late Obliteration

As long as there is some redundant healthy skin with which to work, the Asian blepharoplasty described in Chapters 7 and 8 can be performed either partially or entirely along the width of the eyelid (Figs 13-8 to 13-10). The most common findings at the time of the operation include excessive subdermal scarring and inadequate clearance of the underlying orbicularis oculi muscle, orbital septum, or fat pads (pretarsal or preaponeurotic) along the junction of the pretarsal region and the preaponeurotic space (Fig. 13-11).

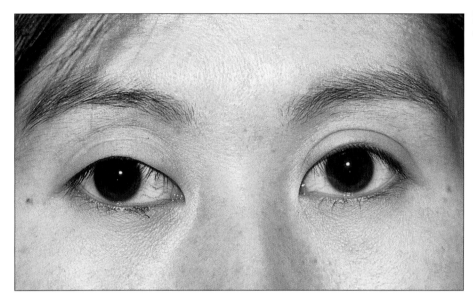

Fig. 13-7 Obliteration of the entire crease over the right upper lid.

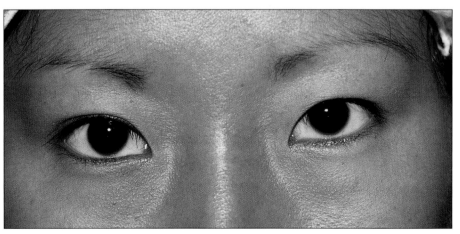

Fig. 13-8 Partially shielded and partially obliterated crease several years after external incision with buried sutures.

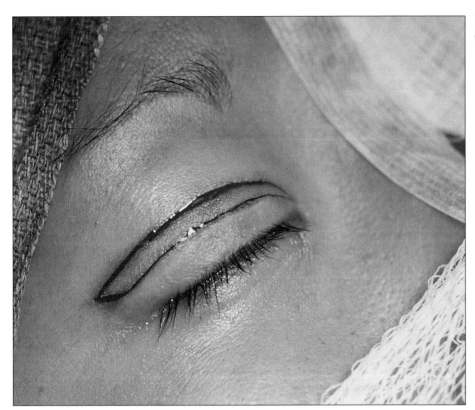

Fig. 13-9 Design of nasally tapered crease. Skin incision has been made.

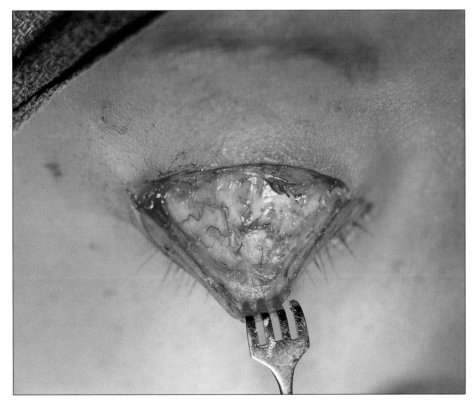

Fig. 13-10 During the operation previously placed levator-to-inferior subcutaneous sutures were an incidental finding.

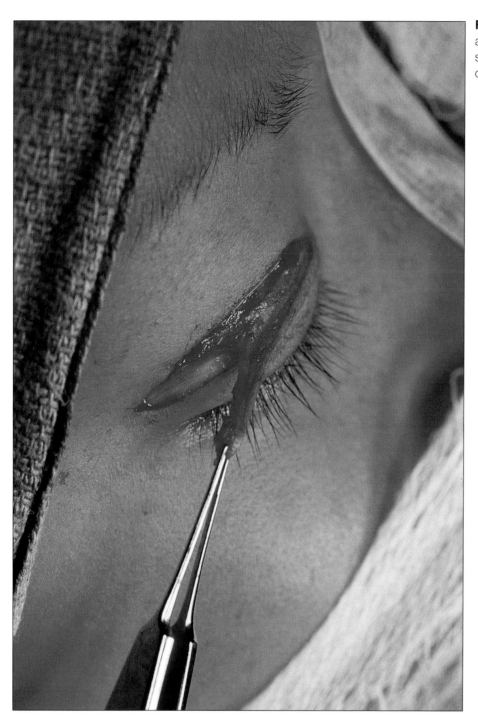

Fig. 13-11 Platform of redundant tissue along the superior tarsal border includes skin, orbicularis muscle, scar tissue, and orbital septum.

Segmental obliteration results in a discontinuous crease, which will fare better if it is completely revised. It is essential to trim away any underlying platform of scar tissue between the skin and the healthy levator aponeurosis along the superior tarsal border. A patient may have an inadequate crease over the medial third (or less) of the upper lid (see Fig. 13-2). This problem is usually the result of insufficient subdermal attachment during the first operation, and can be prevented by using at least three interrupted crease-forming sutures over the medial half of the crease (Fig. 13-12A, B). It may also require more debulking of the underlying soft tissue in that region to allow for solid subcutaneous aponeurotic linkage.

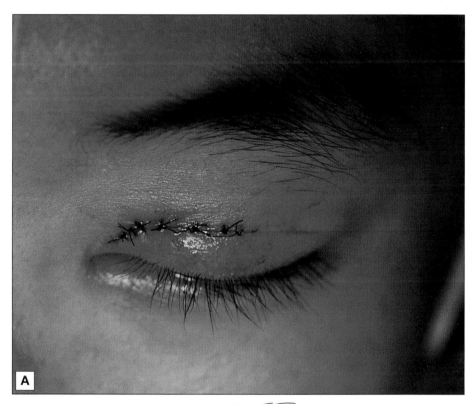

Fig. 13-12 (A, B) Placement of extra interrupted sutures over the medial half of the incision lines in revision for inadequate crease formation over the medial third of the eyelid.

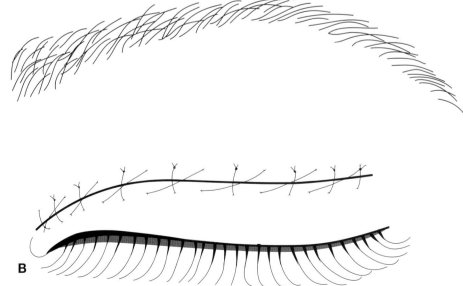

Multiple Creases

Patients may have multiple creases over each eyelid. These can be divided into those who had multiple faint creases to start with, but end up with several competing and prominent creases, and those who were without any crease from the beginning.

Postsurgical Creases Competing with Original Creases

In the first category are patients who may have had several equally rudimentary creases to start with (Fig. 13-13), or who had one noticeable crease with several less obvious ones that became more prominent after surgery. In my experience, this problem is seen in patients who have undergone vigorous dissection in the pretarsal and preaponeurotic spaces (Fig. 13-14), excessive removal of pretarsal tissues in an attempt to remove all pretarsal fat, or overzealous removal of preaponeurotic fat pads. These multiple creases tend to be low and in the pretarsal region.

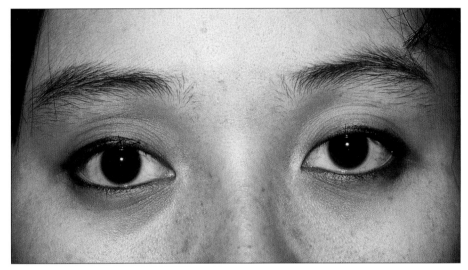

Fig. 13-13 Asian patient with several rudimentary creases.

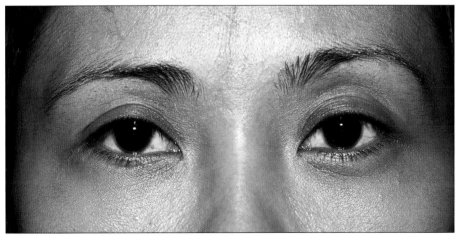

Fig. 13-14 A different Asian patient after blepharoplasty with multiple creases in the pretarsal and supratarsal regions of both lids.

Repair of Multiple Creases

The anatomically based method of Asian blepharoplasty using tarsal height as a guide to crease placement is still the best way to condense several creases into a relatively more dominant one, provided there is enough skin with which to work. Frequently, several closely spaced creases can be completely excised, with good results (see Fig. 15-16). When a patient who presents with multiple creases has a severe shortage of skin, functional correction of the shortage with a full-thickness skin graft takes precedence over the aesthetic repair. The redundant creases may be excised when the skin graft is performed, and a secondary procedure may be performed later to produce a single crease.

Postsurgical Multiple Creases in Patients Without an Original Crease

Almost all multiple creases in the eyelids of patients who did not have a crease to start with result from the excessive removal of preaponeurotic fat pads. These patients frequently had excessively high placement of their main crease, and the redundant creases are all high in the supratarsal region; they are really the interspaces between multiple folds of skin left after the removal of the preaponeurotic fat (see Figs 13-3 and 13-6).

Hollow Supratarsal Sulcus with or without Multiple Creases

An already hollow sulcus may be exaggerated by the removal of preaponeurotic fat, or a hollow sulcus may arise iatrogenically because of the operation.

Repair of Hollow Supratarsal Sulcus

The medical literature contains myriad corrections for a hollow supratarsal sulcus, including the placement of methyl methacrylate implants and the injection of collagen, silicone oil, or free fat globules in the sulcus. The author has not found a good, permanent solution to correcting the problem of excessive removal of preaponeurotic fat. A dermis–fat graft interspaced in the superior conjunctival fornix has been used with some success. In my practice, patients who have a hollow sulcus and multiple folds of redundant skin are given the option of having the folds converted into one crease based on tarsal height.

Semilunar Crease

Patients with a semilunar (half-moon) crease are often unhappy with the result. The primary surgeon may have designed the crease on the basis of the traditional blepharoplasty technique, placing it in such a way that the greatest distance between the crease and the lash margin occurred in the midportion of the eyelid and the ends tapered down toward each canthus. The result is often a round-eyed look. It is especially evident in Asians because they tend to have a narrower eyelid fissure than Caucasians. The same 10-mm separation from crease to lash line, arching toward each canthus, subtends a greater angle in Asians than in Caucasians (Fig. 13-15), hence a greater degree of 'round-eye'. This is the opposite of what most Asians desire. By contrast, a nasally tapered crease with a slight lateral flare or a parallel crease makes the fissure appear wider horizontally, more open-ended, and larger in apparent vertical dimension (Fig. 13-16).

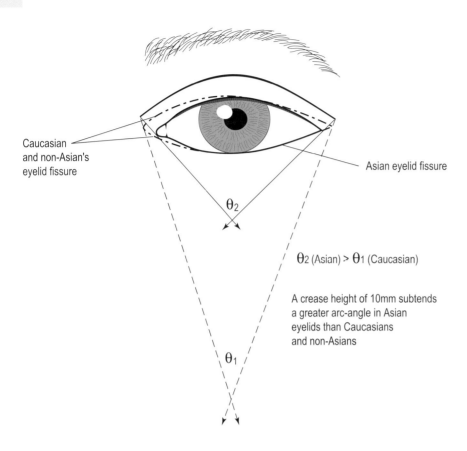

Caucasian
and non-Asian's
eyelid fissure

Asian eyelid fissure

θ_2

θ_2 (Asian) > θ_1 (Caucasian)

A crease height of 10mm subtends
a greater arc-angle in Asian
eyelids than Caucasians
and non-Asians

θ_1

Fig. 13-15 In Asians, a semilunar crease that is 10 mm from the ciliary margin gives an undesirable round-eyed appearance, like Caucasians.

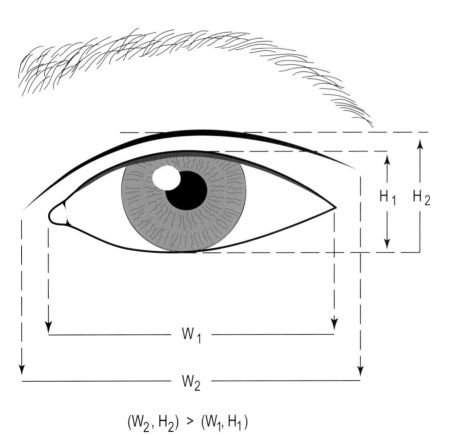

H_1 H_2

W_1

W_2

$(W_2, H_2) > (W_1, H_1)$

Fig. 13-16 In Asians, a nasally tapered or parallel crease gives an open appearance to the eyelid fissures.

Repair of Semilunar Crease

A tarsal height-based technique of Asian blepharoplasty is preferred, utilizing a crease height of 6.5–8.5 mm, with a nasally tapered or parallel configuration. An 'external' skin incision approach allows accurate placement of sutures over the aponeurosis and provides greater control over crease formation.

1. If the maximum height of the crease to be revised is 10 mm or less, the central 50% of the crease may be moved down in the following manner.

1a. For Patients with Some Redundancy of Skin
After 6–9 months from the last operation, the central tarsal height is measured and transcribed on to the eyelid skin. The segment of skin, usually not more than 2–3 mm wide, between this preferred crease line and the undesirable, higher semicircular crease is marked. The central 50% of the semilunar crease is excised, together with the 2-mm strip of skin between it and the preferred lower crease (Fig.

13-17). This maneuver has the effect of converting the crease to a nasally tapered configuration.

A mild degree of undermining is performed along the upper edge of the semilunar crease to free any subcutaneous attachment of septum and levator aponeurosis. The medial 25% of the semilunar crease becomes the nasally tapered portion of the preferred crease. The central 50% is reshaped at a lower level in a parallel continuous crease; the lateral 25% is excised and revised so that it is either parallel or flares slightly upward, by deliberate anchoring higher than it was. This maneuver is facilitated by undermining of the subcutaneous tissue around the lateral canthal region. The challenge arises when there is very little skin between the lateral portion of the semilunar crease and the lateral canthus. I find it effective to excise the lateral 25% of the crease and to perform a simple plastic closure. Six months later I perform a lateral crease revision.

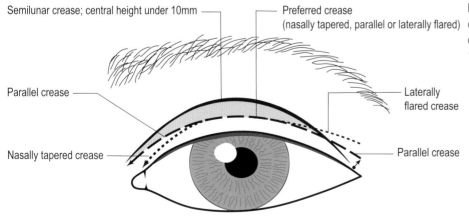

Semilunar crease; central height under 10mm

Preferred crease
(nasally tapered, parallel or laterally flared)

Parallel crease

Laterally
flared crease

Nasally tapered crease

Parallel crease

Fig. 13-17 Design of a nasally tapered or parallel crease in the surgical correction of a semilunar crease within 10 mm of the ciliary margin.

1b. For patients with a shortage of skin A semilunar crease is not easily revised unless the crease, with its underlying scar and the skin between it and the desired new crease (based on tarsal height), is completely excised. A full-thickness graft is used to correct the skin shortage above the proposed crease and to allow for reconstruction of the new crease (Figs 13-18 and 13-19), which will be formed at the junction of the pretarsal skin and the graft.

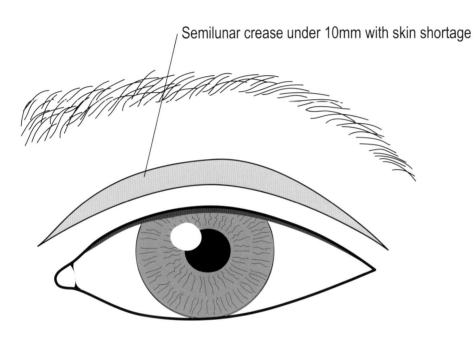

Semilunar crease under 10mm with skin shortage

Fig. 13-18 In the surgical correction of a semilunar crease that is within 10 mm of the ciliary border but in which there is a skin shortage, the scar line of the semilunar crease and the very small segment of pretarsal skin between it and the new crease must be excised (shaded area).

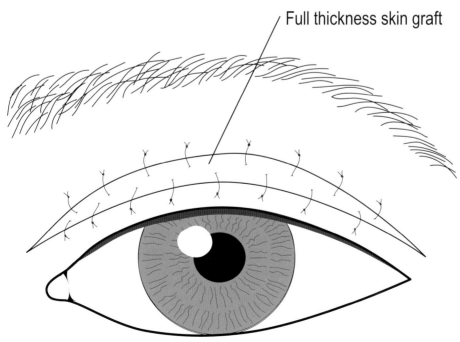

Full thickness skin graft

Fig. 13-19 Full-thickness skin grafting.

2. An extremely challenging situation exists when the semilunar crease is more than 10 mm from the lid margin. I have seen patients with creases as high as 12–14 mm from the margin (Fig. 13-20) (see also Fig. 3-15, and Chapter 3 Unnatural, high, and harsh syndrome). The correction of this involves working closer to the thick dermis of the eyebrow, which provides little camouflage and increases the risk of hypertrophic scarring.

2a. On the rare occasion when there is some redundant skin in conjunction with a highly placed semilunar crease (more than 10 mm from the ciliary margin), one may try the same steps as described for patients with a semilunar crease less than 10 mm (see above).

2b. Unfortunately, most patients whose crease is more than 10 mm from the lid margin have undergone excessive skin removal and have little left for plastic reconstruction. The repair requires a full-thickness skin graft (as above), and the upper edge of the graft will be quite conspicuous (please refer to Chapter 17).

Complete Crease Reversal

The author's most challenging operations have been on the few patients who genuinely wanted their surgically placed crease completely reversed. For these patients I have used a variety of methods, some with better results than others (see Chapter 15, Case 17), and these are rated by me in the next section.

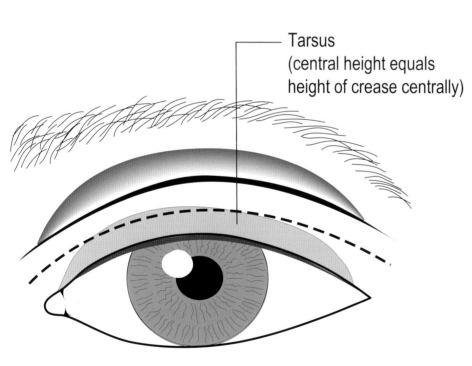

Tarsus
(central height equals
height of crease centrally)

Fig. 13-20 A semilunar crease (solid line) that has been placed more than 10 mm from the ciliary border, almost halfway to the eyebrow for an Asian. The dotted line shows the desired crease, which is based on the central tarsal height. The area above the high, semilunar crease shows a hollow supratarsal sulcus (stippled area), from which fat has been aggressively removed.

Effectiveness of the Corrective Measures to Reverse a Crease

Significant Improvement

Significant improvement is achieved with excision of the crease and scar, and recession of the levator aponeurosis coupled with placement of autologous temporalis fascia or fascia lata.

Some Improvement

1. Some improvement is achieved with excision of the crease and scar, with interposition of pedicled orbicularis muscle fibers to block the aponeurosis–subdermal attachment.
2. Some improvement is also achieved by excising the crease and the scar and applying one-quarter-inch sterile adhesive strips to the sutured skin wound. Patients are encouraged to avoid looking up during the first week after the operation to avoid contraction of the levator aponeurosis.

Minimal Improvement

1. Minimal improvement is achieved with excision of the crease and the scar and the application of traction sutures inferiorly (reverse Frost sutures).
2. Subcutaneous lysis of adhesions using a small tenotomy scissors also usually results in minimal improvement.

As the surgeon acquires expertise, previously unsolvable suboptimal results can be logically analyzed, much as a biochemist analyzes the different factors of a complex reaction. When the different parameters can be clearly and accurately delineated, it may be possible to formulate a plan to correct the problem in a harmonious way. Clearly, the correction should never lead to worsening of the existing problem.

The following is a matrix (Fig. 13-21) with the vertical columns listing suboptimal factors that can occur in the area above the crease, the preseptal (supratarsal) region; and the horizontal rows listing suboptimal factors occuring in the area below the crease, the pretarsal regions. Since suboptimal results seldom occur only in one zone, the surgical solutions listed in each box (cell) shows the correction for the upper preseptal region as well as the lower pretarsal region, with the crease indicated by the dotted line.

Further Reading

1. Expert Commentary on 'Blepharoplasty: special considerations in the Asian eyelid', Chapter 4.7, pp 227–229, in: Mauriello J, ed. Techniques of cosmetic eyelid surgery: a case study approach. Baltimore: Lippincott Williams & Wilkins, 2004.
2. Chen WPD. Management of the eyelid crease: advanced techniques. In: Chen WPD, Khan J, McCord C, eds. Color atlas of cosmetic oculofacial surgery. Oxford: Butterworth–Heinemann, 2004: Chapter 15.

		Preseptal region			
Upper and Lower solutions	**Hollow sulcus**	**Multiple lines**	**Skin shortage**	**Immobile dense skin**	**Cicatrix to levator aponeurosis**
Multiple lines	Add fat	Lyse adhesions, revise into primary crease	Bevelled revision + FTSG	Bevelled revision + FTSG	Correct ptosis
	Revise, reset crease lower	Revise, reset crease	Revise, reset crease	Revise, reset crease	Revise, reset crease
Skin shortage	Add fat	Lyse adhesions, revise into primary crease	Bevelled revision + FTSG	Bevelled revision FTSG	Correct ptosis
	FTSG	FTSG	FTSG	Pretarsal FTSG	FTSG
Scarred platform	Add fat	Lyse adhesions, revise into primary crease	Bevelled revision + FTSG	Bevelled revision + FTSG	Correct ptosis
	Excise, revise vs FTSG	Excise, revise vs FTSG	Excise $^+/-$ FTSG	Excise, revise vs FTSG	Excise, revise vs FTSG
High crease, edema, fullness	Add fat	Lyse adhesions, revise into primary crease	Bevelled revision + FTSG	Bevelled revision + FTSG	Correct ptosis
	Revise/reset crease lower	Revise/reset crease lower	Revise/reset crease lower	Revise/reset crease lower	Revise/reset crease lower

Pretarsal region

Fig. 13-21 Matrix of solutions in revisional blepharoplasty in Asian upper eyelids.

Primary Cases of Asian Blepharoplasty – Before and After

Chapter 14

William P.D. Chen

The following is a series of uneventful Asian blepharoplasties performed for a variety of indications. The patients all followed a highly individualized regimen of instructions, with detailed attention paid to individual personalities and the author's assessment of patient compliance figured in. These photographs show a range of before-and-after changes, with some facial features showing more of an overall change than others. It appears that those patients who are already aesthetically proportional and symmetrical, with ideal anthropomorphic features, are further enhanced by the surgical creation of a crease fold. In almost all individuals the addition of an upper eyelid crease adds to the overall visual impression of a larger palpebral fissure. The most challenging are those with both a pre-existing narrowed horizontal fissure and a shortened vertical lid opening.

The photographs are arranged with my preoperative assessment notes as well as intraoperative findings correlated with the overall assessment for that patient.

Case 1 (Fig. 14-1 A, B)

A 32-year-old man with a rudimentary crease presented for enhancement of the crease (**A**). Examination revealed the presence of a nasally tapered crease.

Asian blepharoplasty was performed, with enhancement of his existing crease (**B**).

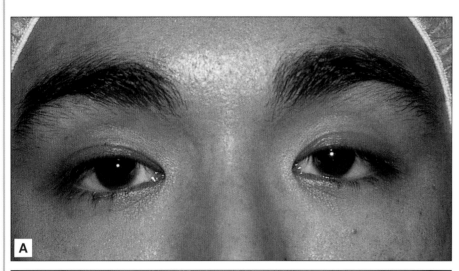

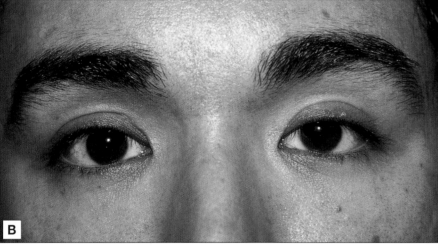

Case 2 (Fig. 14-2 A–C)

A 35-year-old Vietnamese woman presented with an existing nasally tapered crease and a moderate degree of upper lid hooding (**A**). She underwent Asian blepharoplasty, with good results (**B,C**).

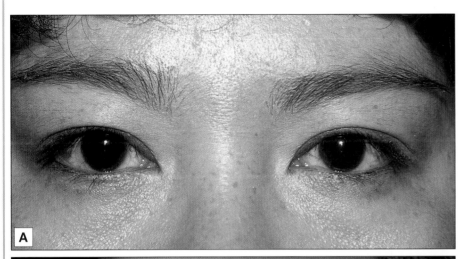

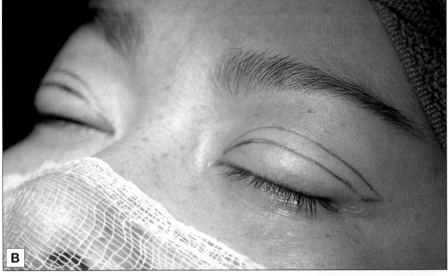

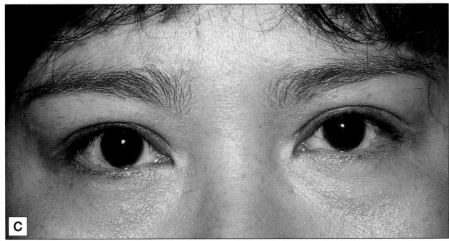

Case 3 (Fig. 14-3 A, B)

A 65-year-old woman who desired a high crease underwent Asian blepharoplasty.

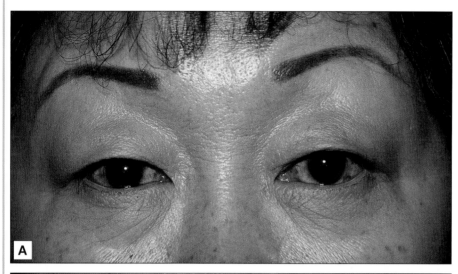

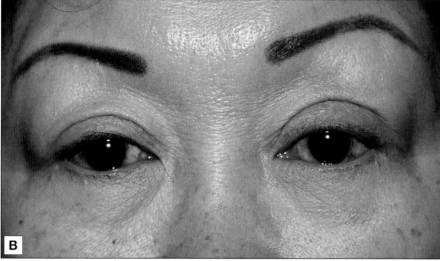

Case 4 (Fig. 14-4 A–C)

The natural upper lid crease of an Asian fashion model. The presence of a nasally tapered crease is noted. The crease does not appear high and is buttressed by a small fold of skin superior to it. (An excessively large fold of skin will result in overhanging and 'shielding' of the crease. 'Shielding' is not to be confused with 'obliteration', where one does not see a distinctive crease even if the fold above it is lifted away.)

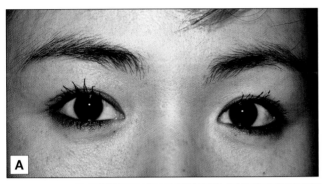

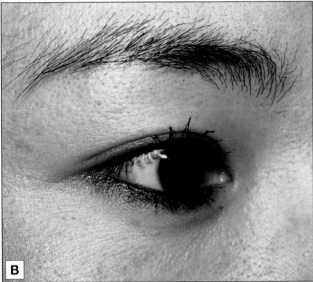

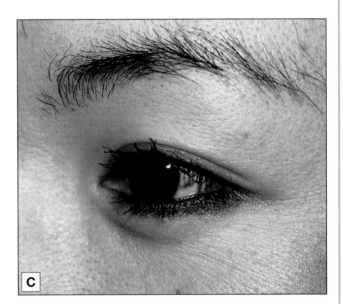

Case 5 (Fig. 14-5 A, B)

Elderly woman for Asian blepharoplasty – note the upper lid hooding and hollowness of the supratarsal sulcus.

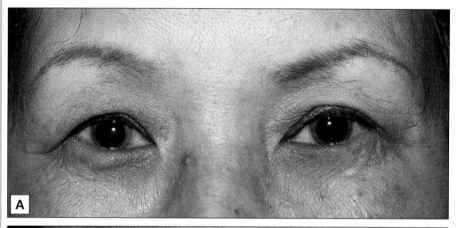

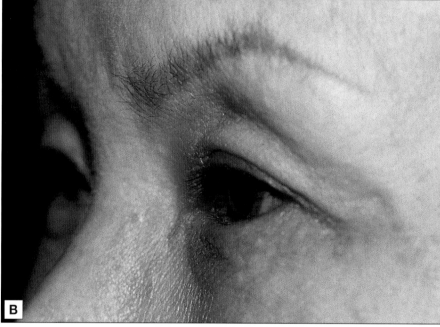

Case 6 (Fig. 14-6 A, B)

A 30-year-old woman with a shielded right upper lid crease and asymmetry of creases. She underwent Asian blepharoplasty with conversion to a parallel crease. She has a minimal 'apparent' bifid crease configuration over the medial end of the right upper crease.

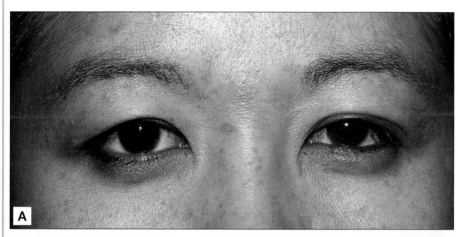

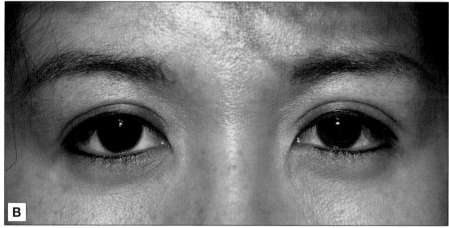

Case 7 (Fig. 14-7 A, B)

A 35-year-old manager with shielding of her natural crease. She underwent Asian blepharoplasty with enhancement of the crease. Preoperative and postoperative views.

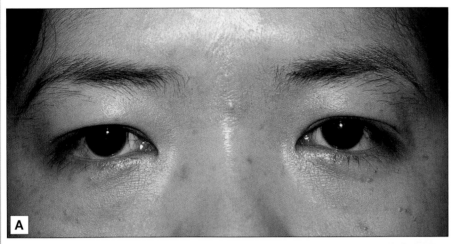

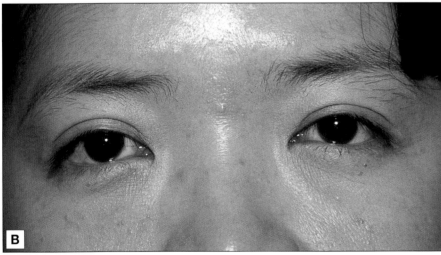

Case 8 (Fig. 14-8 A–C)

(A) A 50-year-old woman with absence of crease. (B) Surgical exploration during Asian blepharoplasty shows an abundance of multiloculated fat pockets in the preaponeurotic as well as the pretarsal plane. (C) The patient 2 months postoperatively (see Appendix 2, Uchida, 1962).

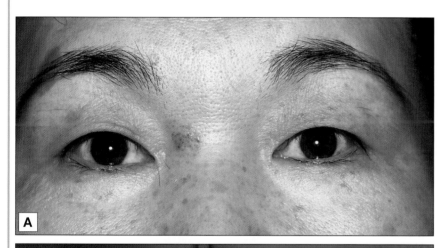

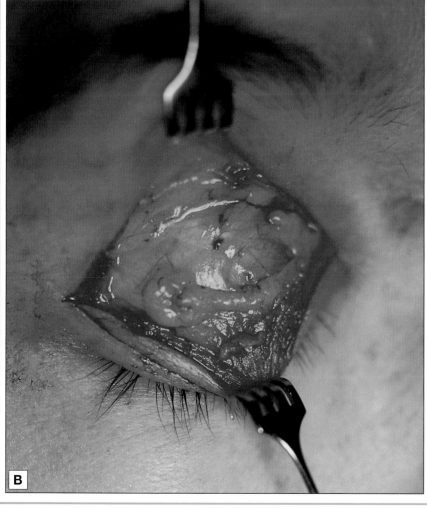

Case 8 (Fig. 14-8 A–C)—cont'd

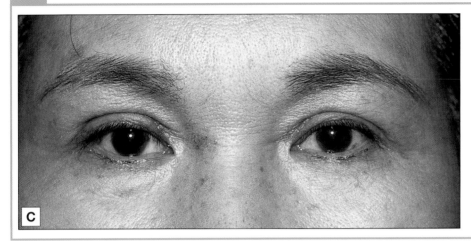

C

Case 9 (Fig. 14-9 A, B)

A 20-year-old female college student with a relatively large face and small eyelid fissure and wide intercanthal distance without a crease. She underwent Asian blepharoplasty with placement of a nasally tapered crease. Preoperative and postoperative views.

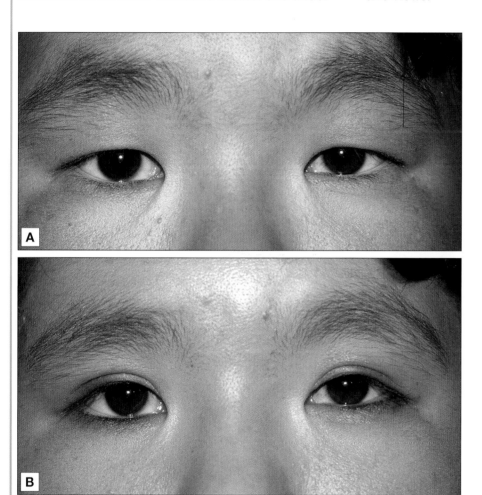

Case 10 (Fig. 14-10 A, B)

A 95-year-old Eurasian (Russian/Chinese) desired upper lid blepharoplasty. Asian blepharoplasty was recommended and performed.

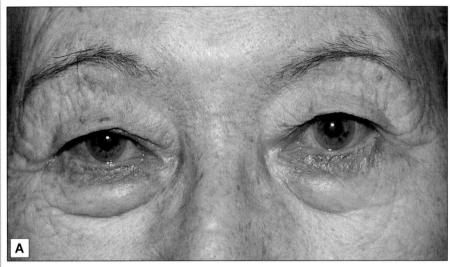

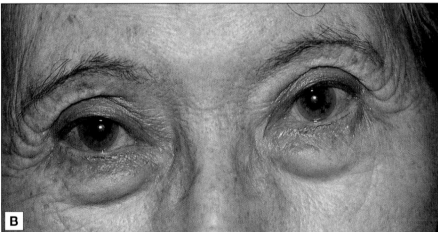

Case 11 (Fig. 14-11 A–D)

(**A**) The presence of a shielded nasally tapered crease over the left upper lid of a 25-year-old woman. (**B**) Pseudo-creases appeared as she looked downward, and faded (**C**) when she looked extremely downward. (**D**) During Asian blepharoplasty, three areas of fat are noted: the pale-yellow and relatively avascular sub-brow (submuscular) fat, the slightly orange-yellowish preaponeurotic fat, which has more blood vessels, and the patchy yellowish pretarsal and sub-cutaneous fat pads. These areas of fat may be present even in an eyelid with a crease.

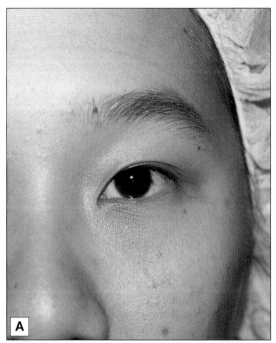

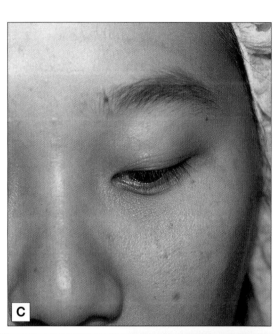

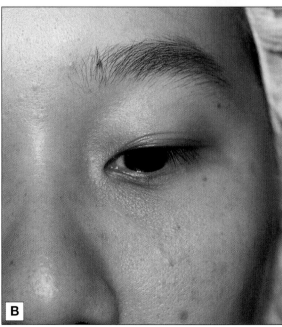

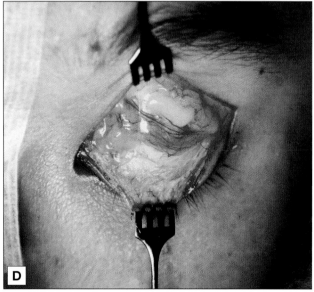

Case 12 (Fig. 14-12 A, B)

A 65-year-old woman who underwent functional Asian blepharoplasty.

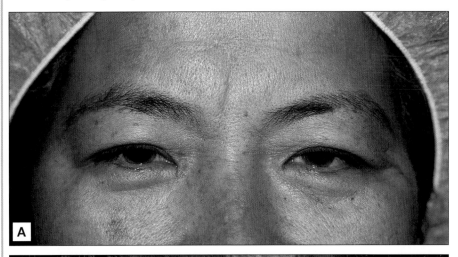

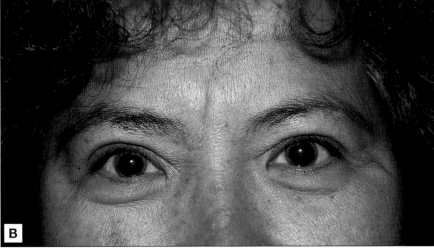

Case 13 (Fig. 14-13 A–E)

A 20-year-old woman with an absent crease (**A**). She underwent Asian blepharoplasty (**B, C**) and clinical photographs were taken 1 week (**D**) and 4 months postoperatively (**E**).

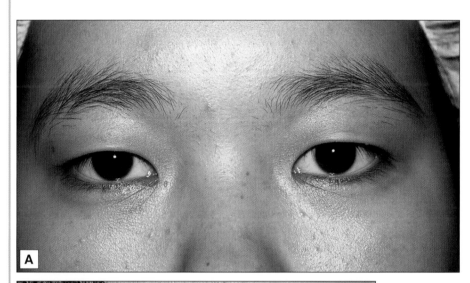

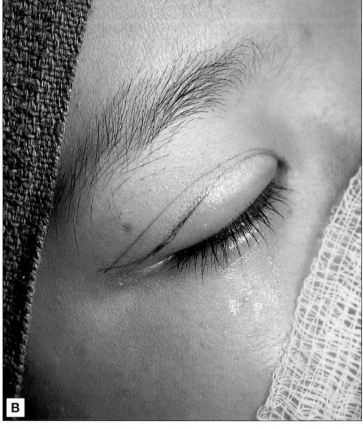

Case 13 (Fig. 14-13 A–E)—cont'd

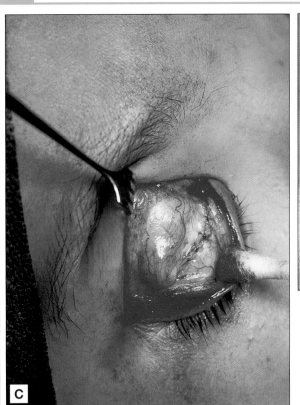

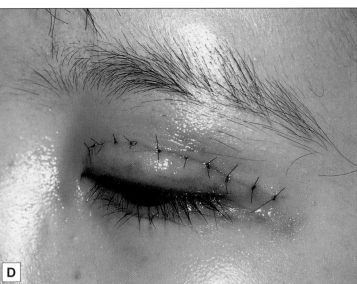

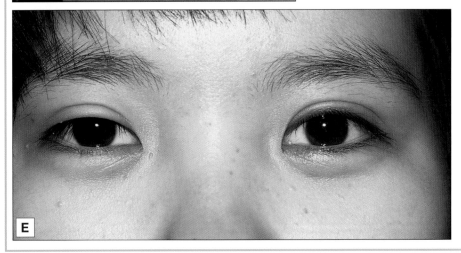

Case 14 (Fig. 14-14 A–G)

(**A**) A 30-year-old fashion model with a partially 'shielded' crease of the right upper lid and a rudimentary crease of the left upper lid (preoperative photograph). (**B**) Postoperatively after Asian blepharoplasty. (**C, D**) The 'dynamic' nature of the crease – distinctive in a straight-ahead view and almost disappearing on downgaze (views taken 1 month postoperatively). (**E**) A year later, the left crease has faded. However, the left crease is still noticeable when she smiles (**F**). (**G**) The left crease was revised and this photograph was taken 9 months after the revision.

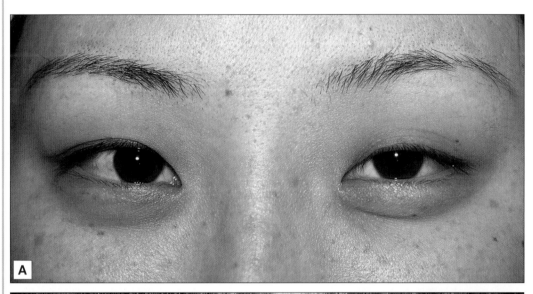

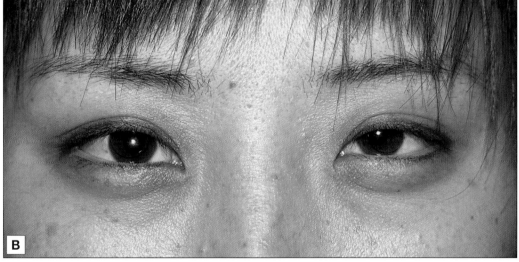

Case 14 (Fig. 14-14 A–G)—cont'd

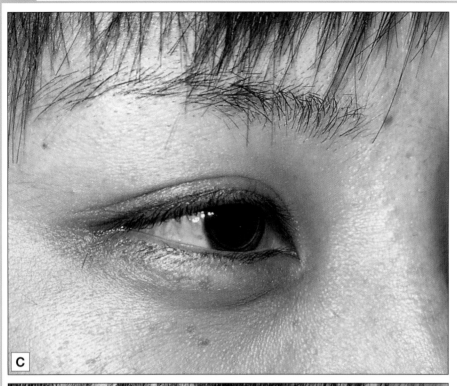

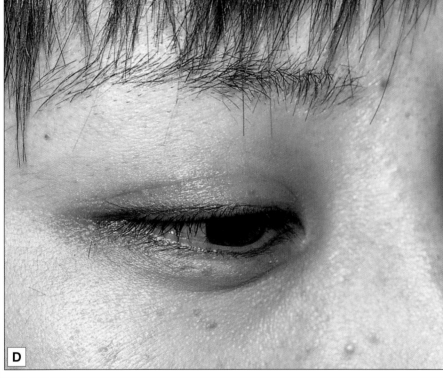

Case 14 (Fig. 14-14 A–G)—cont'd

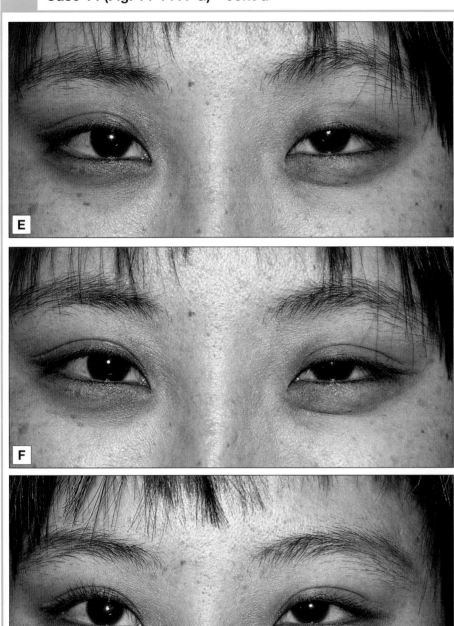

Case 15 (Fig. 14-15 A–C)

(A) A 20-year-old woman with a 'shielded' crease of the right upper lid and absent crease over the left. (B) One week after Asian blepharoplasty. (C) Two months postoperatively. Note the parallel appearance of the crease. It illustrates the downward migration of the crease owing to resolution of tissue edema in the pretarsal region.

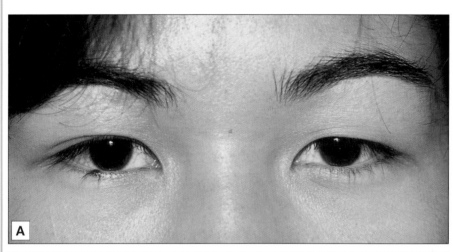

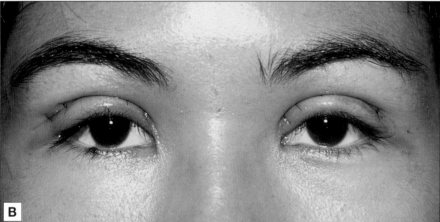

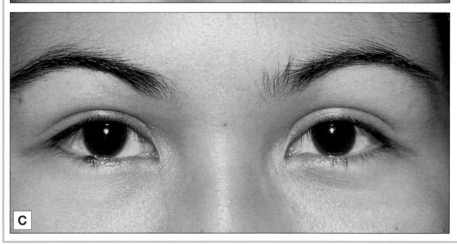

Case 16 (Fig. 14-16 A–C)

(**A**) An 18-year-old woman with absent crease of the right upper lid and mild ptosis. (**B**) Two months after Asian blepharoplasty and ptosis repair – note the distinctive nasally tapered crease merging with the supracanthal fold. (**C**) Two and a half years after surgery.

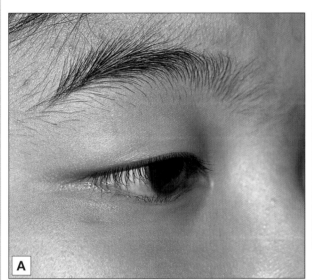

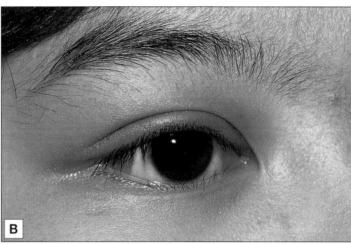

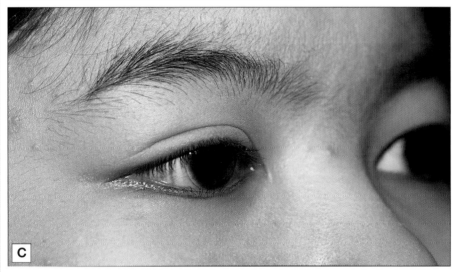

Case 17 (Fig. 14-17 A–C)

A 25-year-old with an absent crease over the right upper lid and a partially shielded crease over the left. Asian blepharoplasty was performed on both sides. At the time of surgery, a large amount of preaponeu-rotic fat pad could be seen over the left upper lid, the side with the crease. Postoperative view was taken 3 weeks later.

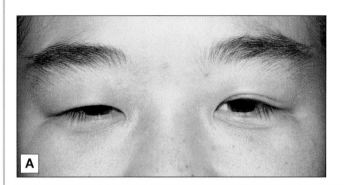

A

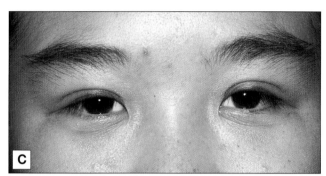

C

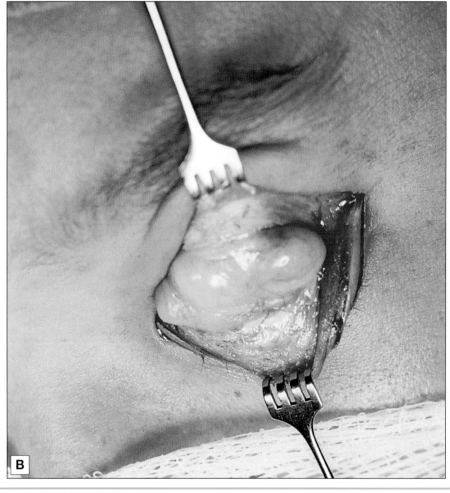

B

Case 18 (Fig. 14-18 A–F)

Steps showing a typical Asian blepharoplasty. (**A**) On the right upper lid the lower line of the lid crease incision is placed according to the measured central height of the tarsus. (**B**) The upper and lower incision is made with a no. 15 blade. (**C**) The orbital septum is opened transversely over the upper edge of the incision. Preaponeurotic fat pads are trimmed appropriately. (**D**) After fat removal. (**E**) A very small amount of the pretarsal and preseptal orbicularis muscles is trimmed (left upper lid). (**F**) The lid crease wound is closed using five to six interrupted 6/0 nylon sutures followed by a continuous 7/0 nylon suture.

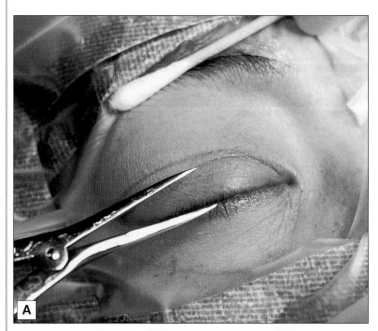

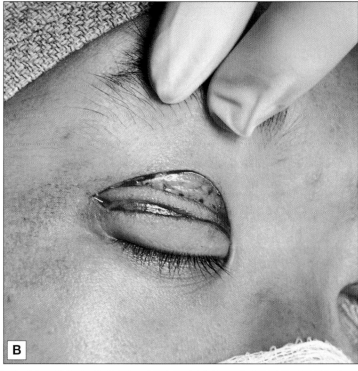

Case 18 (Fig. 14-18 A–F)—cont'd

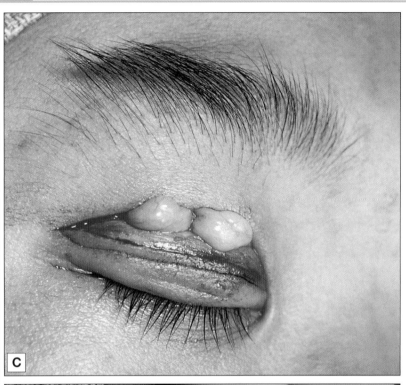

C

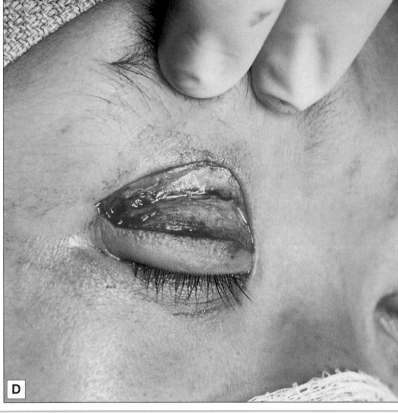

D

Case 18 (Fig. 14-18 A–F)—cont'd

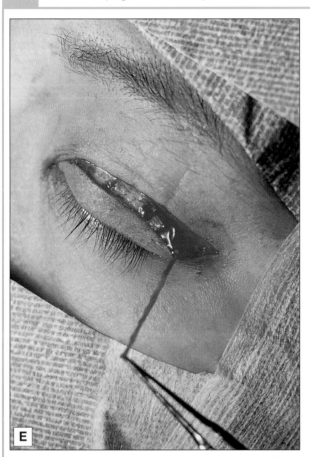

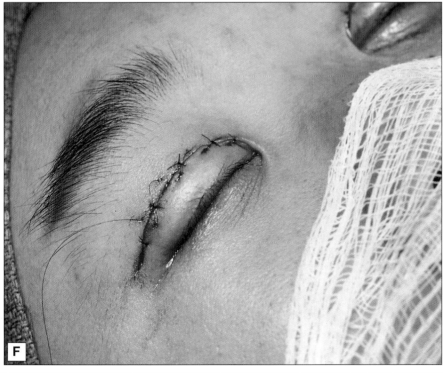

Case 19 (Fig. 14-19 A, B)

(A) A 55-year-old woman with a rudimentary crease on the right upper lid. (B) During surgical exploration the right upper lid showed a lower point of fusion of the orbital septum, all the way down to the pretarsal region. Fat pads were noted in the preseptal and pretarsal regions.

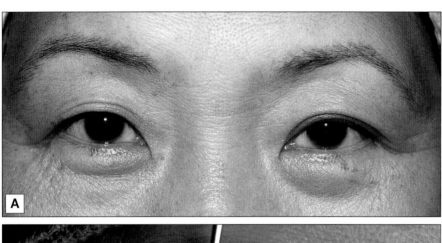

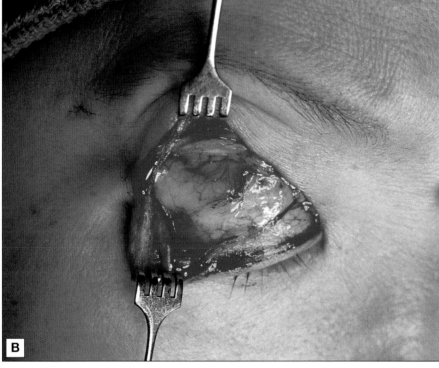

Case 20 (Fig. 14-20 A–F)

(**A**) A 30-year-old patient; preoperative views. (**B**) Postoperatively following Asian blepharoplasty. (**C, D**) Left upper lid before-and-after views. (**E, F**) Right upper lid before-and-after views.

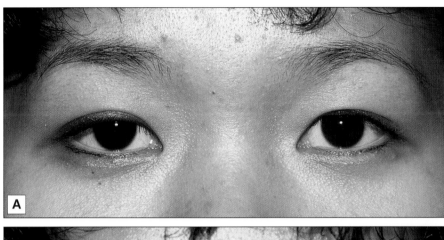

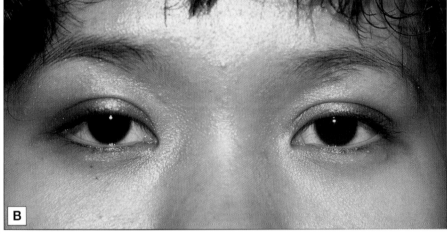

Case 20 (Fig. 14-20 A–F)—cont'd

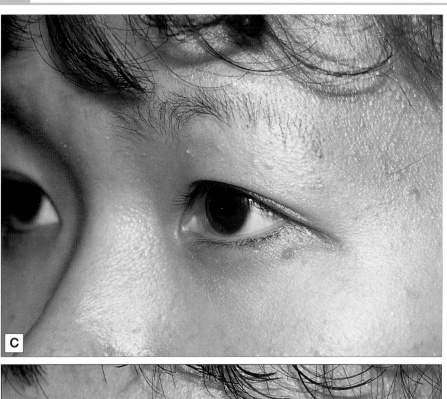

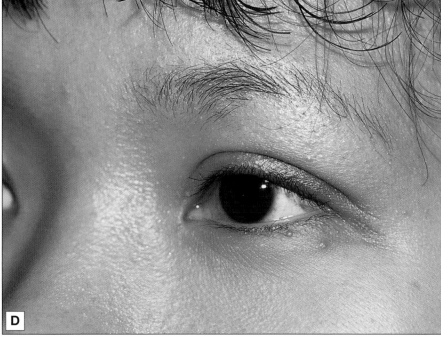

Case 20 (Fig. 14-20 A–F)—cont'd

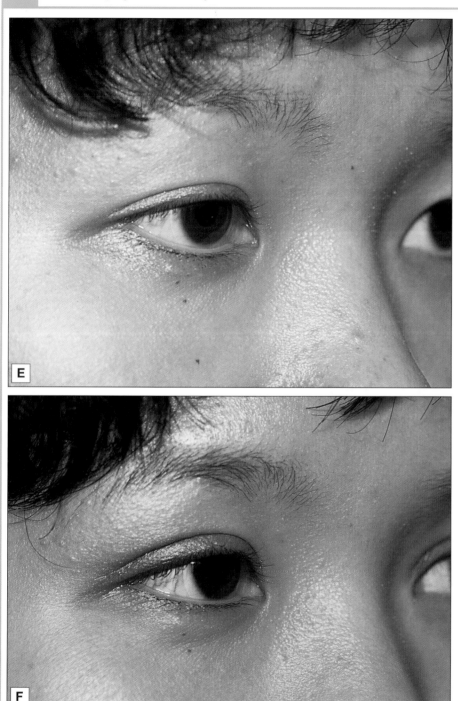

Case 21 (Fig. 14-21 A–C)

(A) A patient with absence of a crease over the right upper lid. (B) Two months after Asian blepharoplasty; minimal edema is still present. (The patient is fixing his gaze on the camera's flash unit on top rather than at the lens aperture.) (C) Appearance 4 months postoperatively.

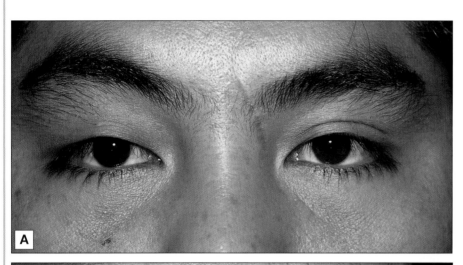

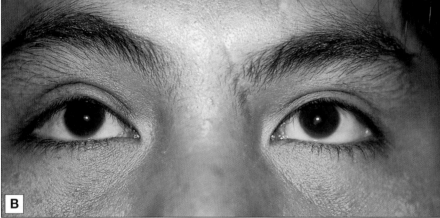

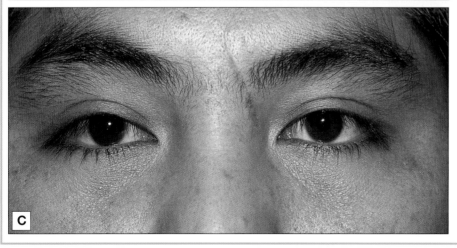

Case 22 (Fig. 14-22 A, B)

26F with heavy fat pads laterally, slightly triangular, and a small fissure. Wants a low-set NTC.

I/O (intraoperatively): tarsus 6.5 mm. Had a heavy bed of fat overlying along the superior tarsal border. Required a U-shaped 'square well' debulking of the fat overlying the STB (superior tarsel border); excised lateral preaponeurotic fat, and reduced sub-brow fat.

For a right-handed surgeon the tendency is to excise the myocutaneous strip of the right upper eyelid starting from thc latcral end; this has a tendency to be shallow laterally as you proceed medially, therefore more tissue is left behind laterally and there is a higher likelihood of partial obliteration (regression) of the crease there.

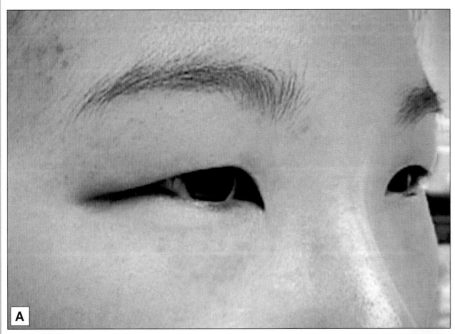

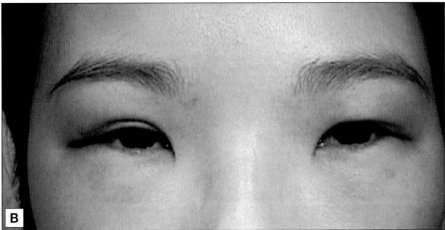

Case 23 (Fig. 14-23 A–C)

20F, single lid, with lateral two-thirds hooding. The patient desired a parallel crease (**A**).

I/O: tarsus 8 mm. As she was 5′2″ tall I used 7 mm in designing a parallel crease. Most of the pre-aponeurotic fat was excised. (**B**) Ten months later the RUL (right upper lid) crease had not formed well, the LUL (left upper lid) was perfect and parallel.

(**C**) Postoperatively following crease enhancement on right upper lid.

During the touch-up enhancement I designed a 7 mm parallel line +1.5 mm, which included the old scar. Excised M/C strip of scarred skin. Levator appeared thin for her age, although she was without ptosis and had excellent levator function. Some fatty tissue over the medial extent of the parallel crease was excised to help the infolding. Multiple 6/0 interrupted sutures were applied for crease construction.

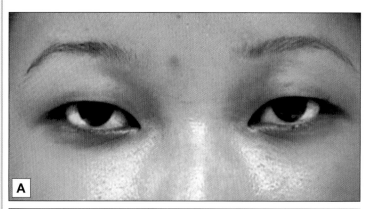

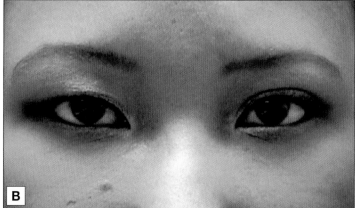

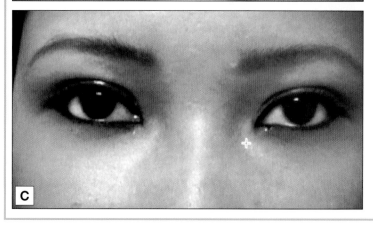

Case 24 (Fig. 14-24 A, B)

18M, 5'7". Rudimentary crease OD (right eye), has distinct NTC, LUL.

I/O: tarsus 7.5 mm. The rudimentary crease of RUL measured 7 mm. Designed NTC at 7 mm + 2 mm skin. Reduced fat; excised orbicularis overlying along the STB. Medially there was a small web – this was excised and deep placed 6/0 suture through skin as well as orbicularis to form crease without a medial canthal web.

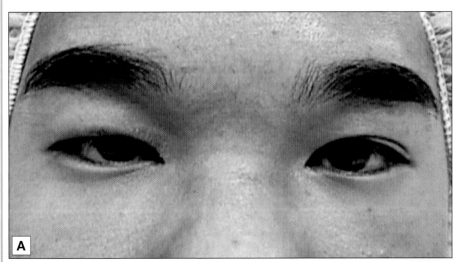

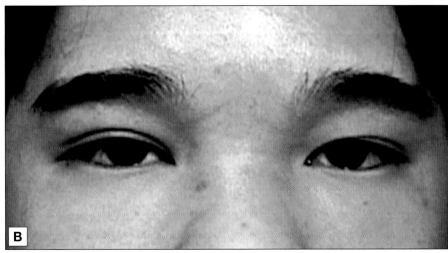

Case 25 (Fig. 14-25 A, B)

43F, 5'4". Wanted parallel crease. Had more skin over RUL and OD fissure smaller size. LUL has a higher pseudocrease.

I/O: used hyaluronidase with 2% xylocaine. Tarsus measured 8 mm. Designed 8 mm parallel crease. Over RUL removed 5 mm segment of skin. Fat untouched. Upon closure of wound, crease now measured at 6 mm. Therefore, redrew LUL crease to be at 6.5 mm, and this side remained unchanged after the procedure.

Conclusion: Hyaluronidase can expand tissue plane and spread out the skin such that 8 mm marking in reality covered 6 mm of skin. The second eye, LUL done 30 minutes later showed no variation in crease position with closure of wound.

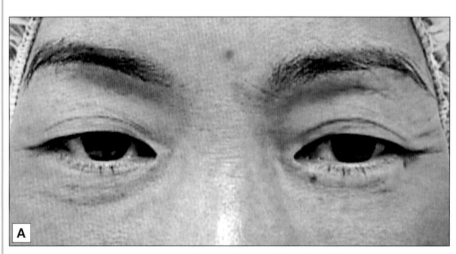

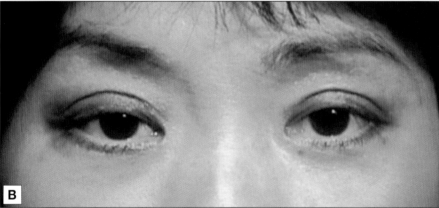

Case 26 (Fig. 14-26)

24F born without crease, but 'developed' mild NTC OD, and hooded and low-set NTC OS. For crease enhancement.

I/O: 7.5 mm tarsus.

RUL designed 7.5 mm crease + 2 mm redundancy; excised inferior orbicularis strip and fatty infiltrate.

Beware of fixating crease along a dehisced edge of the levator aponeurosis as it will probably lead to a higher than expected crease. Should stay along superior tarsal border.

LUL same finding as RUL.

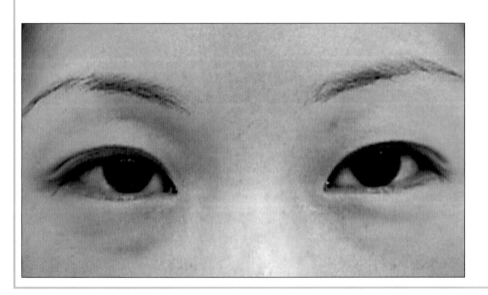

Case 27 (Fig. 14-27 A, B)

57F, slight ptosis RUL, covers 2 mm cornea. Heavy edematous RUL, moderately heavy LUL. Small fissures OU. Heavy brows.

I/O: I was not able to evert tarsal plate to measure it. Designed 7 mm parallel crease. Found large amount of amorphous fibro-mosaic fat inferiorly to pre- aponeurotic fat (which itself was inferiorly placed). Excised fat. Reinforced the usual crease fixation sutures of 6/0 silk with one double-armed 6/0 Vicryl suture, applied from pretarsal skin to aponeurosis to pretarsal skin.

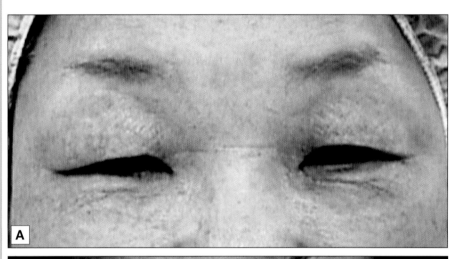

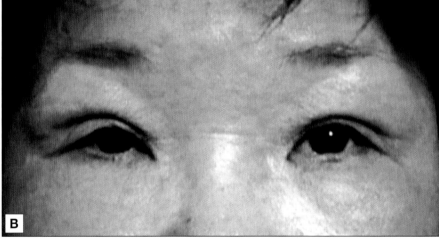

Case 28 (Fig. 14-28 A, B)

23F absent crease, smaller fissure OD, 5′0″, prefers parallel crease. Had mild medial canthal fold (**A**).

I/O: tarsus floppy and measured 6 mm only. Designed 6 mm parallel crease.

RUL had large sheet of amorphous preaponeurotic fat, down to below the superior tarsal border. This was dissected off of the underlying shiny healthy aponeurosis, and excised. Excised larger than usual amount of myocutaneous strip, which appeared boggy from fatty infiltration of the orbicularis muscle.

Treatment of Medial Canthal Fold

Small redundant of 'dog-ear' over the medial end of the crease wound is based along the lower border. It was overlapped onto the upper skin edge and excised appropriately. The two edges are then anchored with 6/0 silk. The bite along the upper skin edge is exaggerated in terms of the amount of skin taken as well as the depth of the orbicularis that is secured. The knot is pulled and tied onto the upper side of the wound. It will then heal imperceptibly, as the edges are perfectly aligned and without tension.

LUL: also excised larger strip of mycocutaneous tissues. Medial dog-ear similarly treated.

(**B**) One week postoperative appearance.

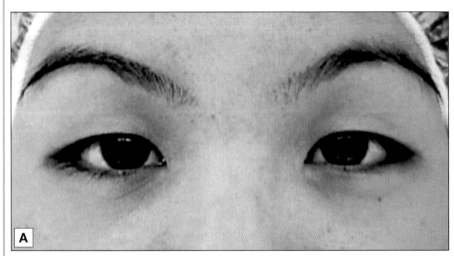

A

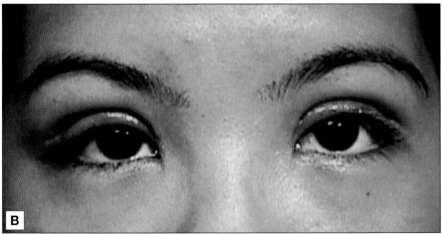

B

Case 29 (Fig. 14-29 A, B)

22F, intermittent creasing over RUL, LUL never creases and has smaller fissure. Prefers parallel crease with lateral flare. Levator function OD 9mm, OS 12–13mm. 5'3" (A).

I/O: tarsus 8mm. Designed minimally tapering parallel crease, plus 2mm redundancy. Excised moderate amount of preaponeurotic fat that migrated over the STB, although it was not apparent clinically on preoperative examination. Excised M/C strip.

(B) One week postoperative appearance.

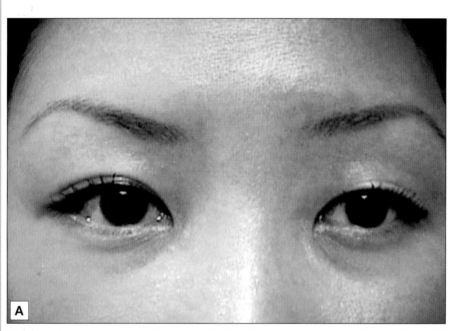

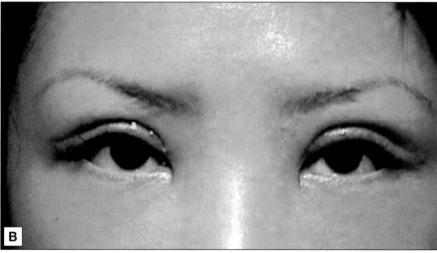

Case 30 (Fig. 14-30)

34F with mild lid retraction. Upper lid margin at superior corneal limbus. Had rudimentary multiple partial lines OU. Wanted NTC. 5′3″.

I/O: tarsus 9 mm. Used 7 mm and designed NTC, + 2 mm skin. RUL has 3+ fat over lateral 2/3 of lid, LUL 2+ fat lateral 2/3 of lid. The inferior orbicularis was very vascular over the lateral end of the incision.

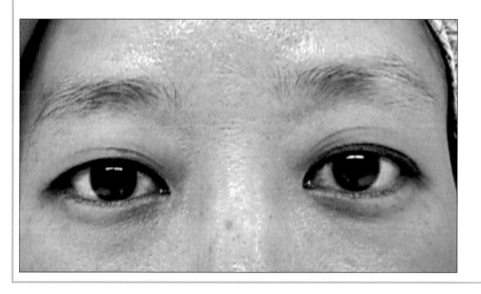

Case 31 (Fig. 14-31 A, B)

27F, high brows, moderate fat OU, large eyes with OS being larger. 5′7″. Desires NTC.

I/O: designed 6.5 mm NTC OU. Found amorphous fat and preaponeurotic fat close to STB; they were reduced. Also excised a strip of fibroadipose tissue along the anterior aspect of the STB. Formed crease with 6/0 and 7/0 silk.

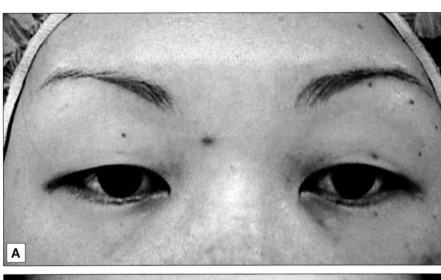

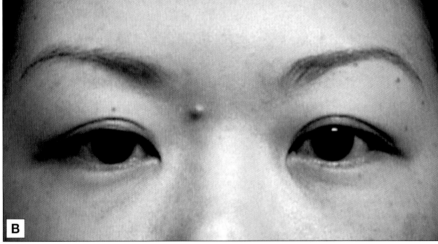

Case 32 (Fig. 14-32 A, B)

28F absent crease, desires low-set NTC. 5′3″. Had severe brow overaction with some head-tilt backward position (**A**).

I/O: tarsus 8 mm. Designed 7.5 mm + 2 mm skin redundancy. Had prominent preaponeurotic fat requiring excision OU. Had abundant soft, mosaic tissue redundancy along the STB which was excised.

(**B**) One week postoperative appearance.

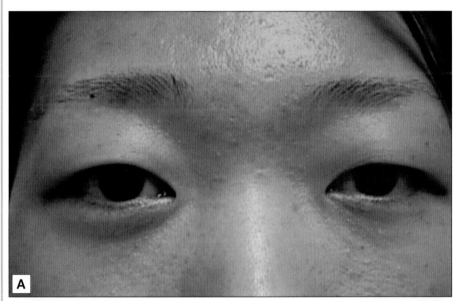

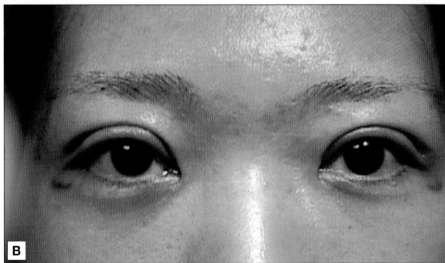

Case 33 (Fig. 14-33 A, B)

23F wears lid crease tape constantly for her RUL, and occasionally for LUL. Has hooded shielded skin over lateral RUL, and incomplete non-joining crease lines over lateral pretarsal area of LUL. Prefers NTC (**A**).

I/O: tarsus 7.5 mm. Designed 7 mm NTC.

RUL: reduced significant preaponeurotic fat; excised a band of fibroadipose tissue along the STB.

LUL: rechecked drawn crease to ensure it is 7 mm. Same procedure as RUL.

(**B**) One week postoperative appearance.

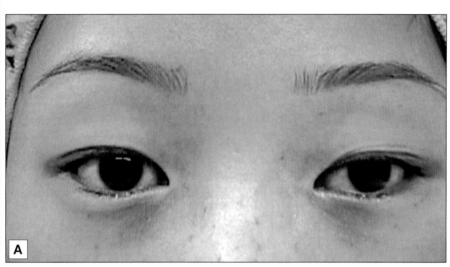

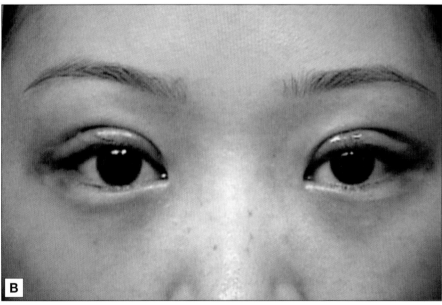

Case 34 (Fig. 14-34 A, B)

28F, uses lid crease tape and make-up to help crease formation. Pretarsal skin is pink from taping. Desires parallel crease (**A**).

I/O: tarsus 8.5 mm. Designed 7.5 mm parallel crease. Preaponeurotic fat appeared fibrotic and inferiorly located. Reduced with Wetfield bipolar cautery.

Mycocutaneous strip, which was very vascular, was excised. The crease may look broader on one side than the other during the immediate healing period due to hematoma.

(**B**) One week postoperative appearance.

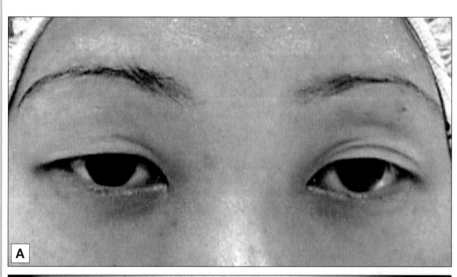

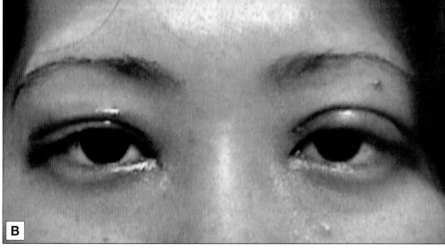

Case 35 (Fig. 14-35 A, B)

25M absent crease. Triangular hooding. Prefers NTC with average crease height. 5′10″ (**A**).

I/O: tarsus 7.5 mm. Designed 7 mm NTC. There was no preaponeurotic fat. Cleared preaponeurotic platform. Formed crease.

(**B**) One week postoperative appearance.

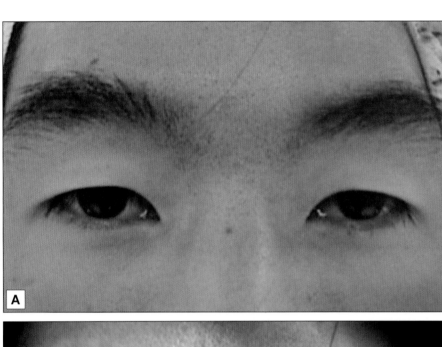

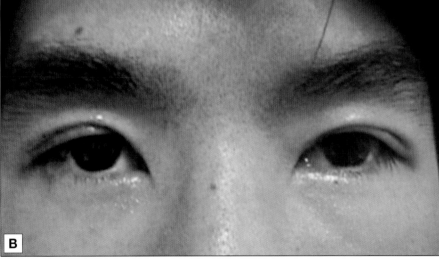

Case 36 (Fig. 14-36 A, B)

35F Upper lid hooding with shielded NTC. Desired a more prominent crease. 5′5″.

I/O: tarsus 7.5 mm. Designed same 7.5 mm NTC + 2 mm skin. (Beware of tendency of right-handed surgeon or right-eye dominant individual to mark the LUL crease's lateral extent shorter than it should be. Always compare both sides.)

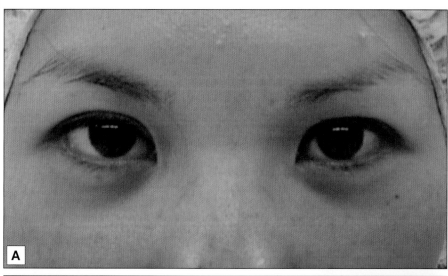

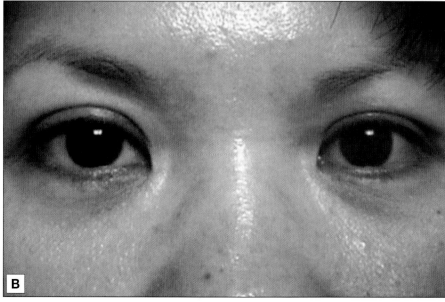

Case 37 (Fig. 14-37 A, B)

18F absent crease with mild ptosis, more over the left side. Desires standard height NTC. 5'3".

I/O: tarsus 8 mm. Designed 7.5 mm NTC. Removed fraction of fat. Had to lyze some adhesion between the inferior skin edge and orbicularis to the aponeurosis along the STB, in order to better place the 6/0 silk.

LUL: medial canthal dog-ear treated with direct excision of inferior dog-ear and supraplacement of suture knot.

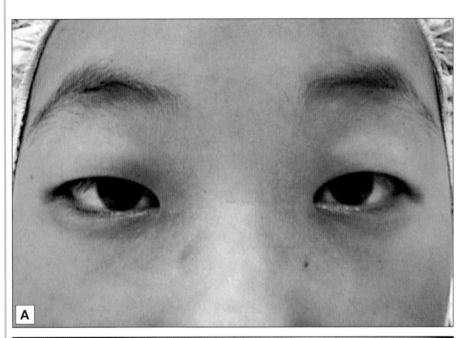

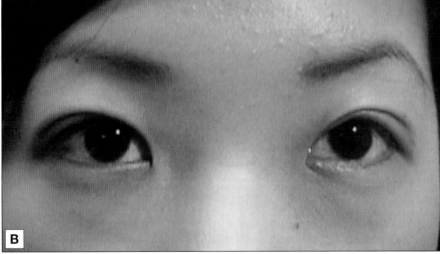

Case 38 (Fig. 14-38)

21F absent crease, with medial canthal fold. Prefers parallel crease with average height.

I/O: tarsus 7 mm. Designed 7 mm parallel crease. Large amount of inferiorly migrated preaponeurotic fat was reduced with bipolar cautery. Large roll of subcutaneous intraorbicularis fat along the STB was excised. Used multiple 6/0 interrupted sutures to enhance crease construction.

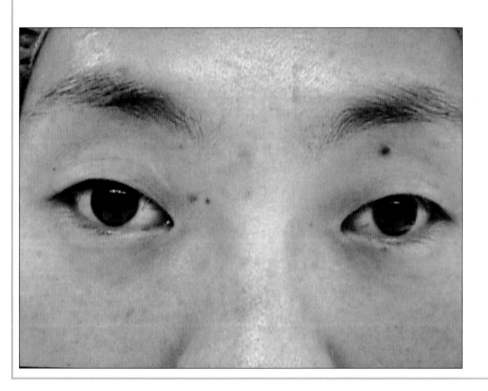

Case 39 (Fig. 14-39 A, B)

26F, RUL has no crease, LUL has a shallow low pseudo-crease line at 3 mm from lashes. 5'4". Desires NTC (**A**).

I/O: tarsus 7 mm. Designed 7 mm NTC + 2 mm skin. Partial excision of preaponeurotic fat OU.

(**B**) RUL formed crease well.

LUL medial half required additional reinforcement with 6/0 interrupted sutures.

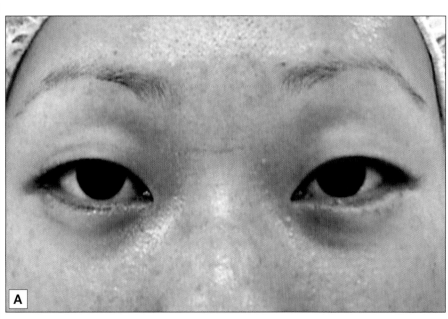

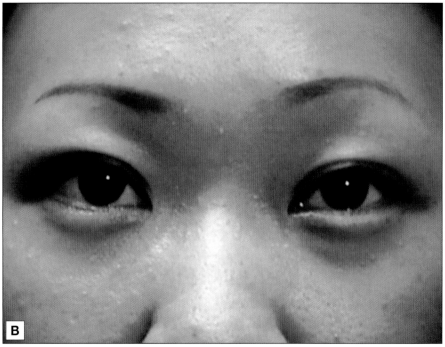

Case 40 (Fig. 14-40 A, B)

19F, uses glue over pretarsal skin for crease formation. Heavily hooded lid with fat. 5′5″. Prefers NTC (**A**).

I/O: tarsus 7.5 mm. Designed 7 mm NTC OU + 2 mm skin. Used beveled approach to orbital septum.

RUL had abundant fat which required partial excision. Formed crease at 7 mm.

LUL: also excised part of fat. The crease thus formed appeared shifted down to 6.5 mm. This could be due to different amount of fat excision between the two sides, and the subsequent change in skin tension as fat has been reduced.

(**B**) One week postoperative appearance.

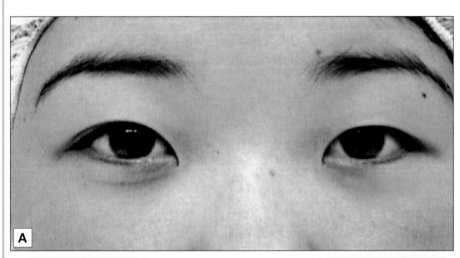

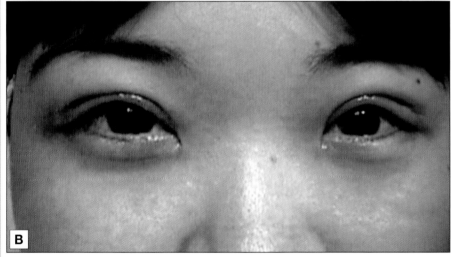

Case 41 (Fig. 14-41)

30F, absent crease OU. Prefers NTC with standard height. 5'7".

I/O: tarsus 8 mm. Used 7 mm to draw NTC + 3 mm skin. No fat was removed. The orbital septum was observed to be fused to the levator aponeurosis in a very ill-defined manner. Had to delineate the superior tarsal border by using the cutting cautery to create a 'mini-trough' over and along the superior tarsal border, then attached multiple 6/0 fixation sutures. Worked well.

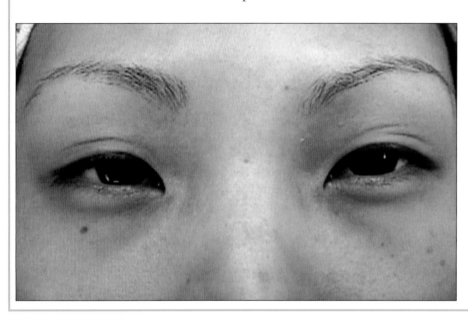

Case 42 (Fig. 14-42 A–C)

24F, 5′2″. Before Asian crease procedure by this author. (**A**) Preoperative appearance.

LUL has a residual skin fold above the original crease incision, which gives the appearance of two crease lines.

(**B**) Appearance following first procedure.

Revision I/O: tarsus 7 mm. Designed 7 mm NTC and included 1.5 mm skin-scar. Bevelled approach along the upper edge toward the preaponeurotic space. Found preaponeurotic fat, which appeared almost untouched, though I knew I had partially excised it before. Excised M/C strip and some redundant fibroadipose tissue along the STB. Formed crease. (**C**) Postoperative appearance following revision enhancement of left upper lid.

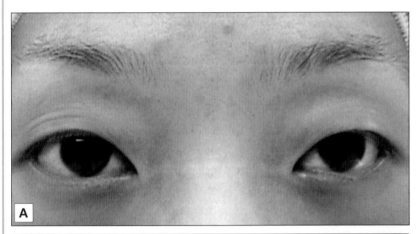

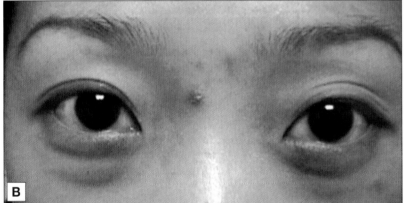

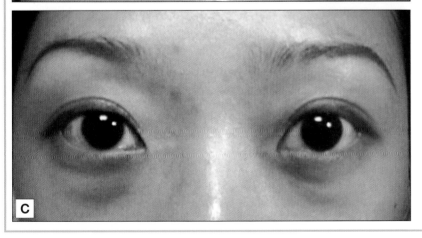

Case 43 (Fig. 14-43 A–C)

35M heavy eyelid with fat bulge. Hooding appears to cover 4 mm of cornea, but lid margin is actually 2 mm on to cornea. 5′5″. Prefers NTC (A).

I/O: tarsus 9.0 mm. During the first procedure I used 7 mm to design NTC. Thick skin with amorphous orbicularis, orbital septum and very little preaponeurotic fat. Formed crease with 6/0 silk and 7/0 silk.

(B) RUL crease obliterated at 6 months and required enhancement.

I/O (revision): boggy lid tissue with amorphous infiltrated fat over the preaponeurotic space as well as within levator itself. These were left untouched. Excised M/C strip that included scarred tissues; created mini-trough along STB. Formed crease with 6/0 and 7/0 sutures. (C) One week postoperative appearance.

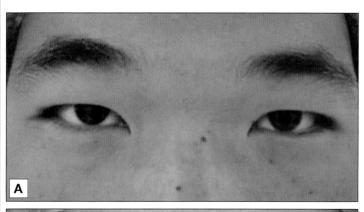

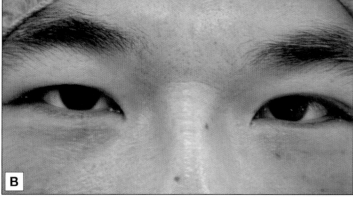

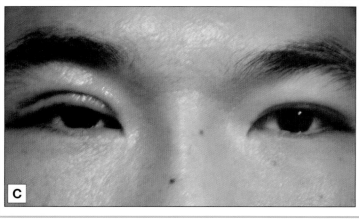

Case 44 (Fig. 14-44 A, B)

23F, uses nail file to manipulate eyelid skin to form crease. Multiple rudimentary crease lines. Prefers parallel crease on her highest crease line.

I/O: tarsus 7 mm. Designed 7.5 mm parallel crease + 2.5 mm skin redundancy. Little fat. Excised M/C strip. Formed crease.

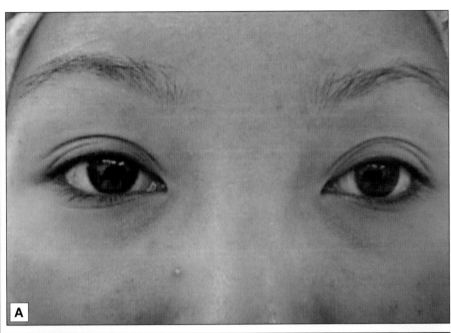

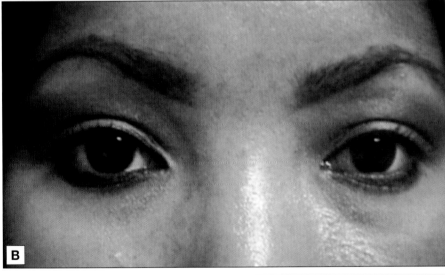

Case 45 (Fig. 14-45 A, B)

34F, Chinese/Hawaiian, 5'4". RUL has hooded NTC. LUL has sulcus above multiple rudimentary creases. Very tanned skin (**A**).

I/O: tarsus 6.5–7mm.

RUL included 2mm skin, LUL + 3mm skin. Has very thin skin, very vascular orbicularis. Both sides had very little preaponeurotic fat and appeared bound down; these were released and repositioned superiorly. Good crease formation.

(**B**) Postoperative appearance (patient wearing colored contact lenses).

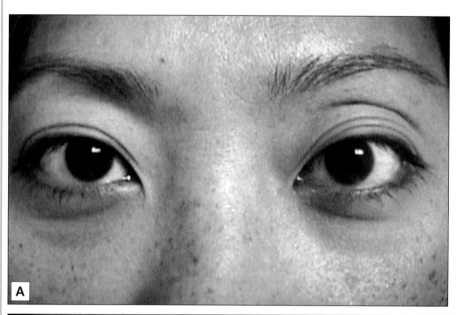

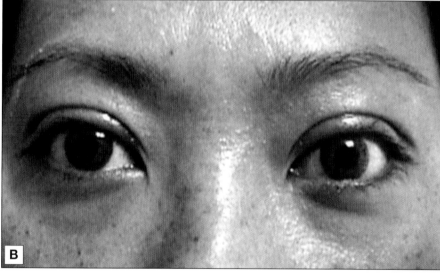

Case 46 (Fig. 14-46)

30F, has no crease RUL, LUL has occasional crease. Prefers above average parallel crease OU.

I/O: tarsus 8.5 mm. Designed 7.5 mm (7 + 0.5) parallel crease line with 2 mm skin.

RUL: preaponeurotic fat very soft, repositioned superiorly. Orbicularis was vascular. Excised M/C strip.

LUL: preaponeurotic fat plastered down over lateral half of aponeurosis; vascular and therefore left alone.

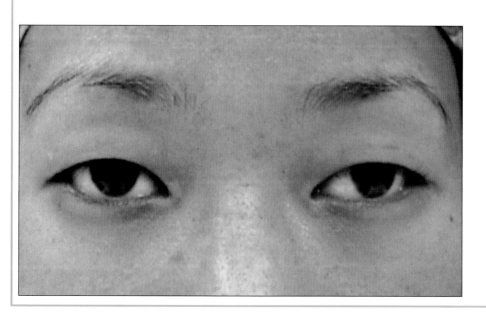

Case 47 (Fig. 14-47 A, B)

22F, 5'7". She had a single lid up until 16 years old. Now has incomplete or partial creases. Used tape daily (**A**).

I/O: tarsus 7.5 mm. Designed 8 mm parallel crease as the lid was edematous from xylocaine. Included 2 mm skin in myocutaneous strip. Orbicularis was very spongy and vascular. Used superiorly beveled approach through septum. The preaponeurotic fat appeared bound down over the lateral half. This was released and repositioned superiorly. Excised M/C strip and inferior orbicularis edge of right side. Formed crease.

(**B**) One week postoperative appearance.

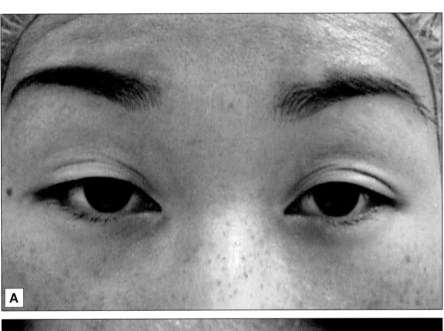

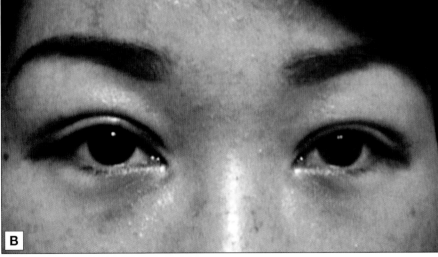

Case 48 (Fig. 14-48)

22M absent crease OU. Left fissure appears larger than right. Desired low-set parallel crease.

I/O: tarsus 8.5 mm. Used 7 mm design for parallel crease. Very vascular over orbicularis. Little pre- aponeurotic fat. Excised M/C flap but did not vigor- ously debulk preaponeurotic platform. Used eight 6/0 silk sutures for crease construction, plus 7/0 silk running stitch.

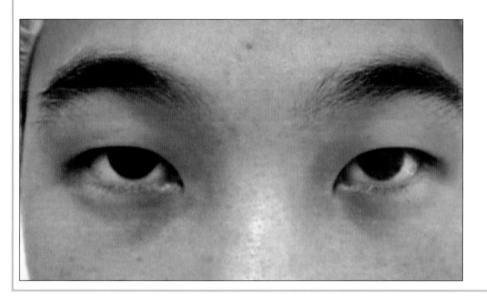

Case 49 (Fig. 14-49 A, B)

31M with absent crease. Heavy lids, large face. 5′10″ (**A**).

I/O: tarsus 8.5 mm. Designed 7 mm parallel crease. Skin very thin and stretched; orbicularis was vascular, with fibromosaic preaponeurotic fat plastered down. Excised around 3.5 mm M/C strip. Crease formed well.

(**B**) One week postoperative appearance.

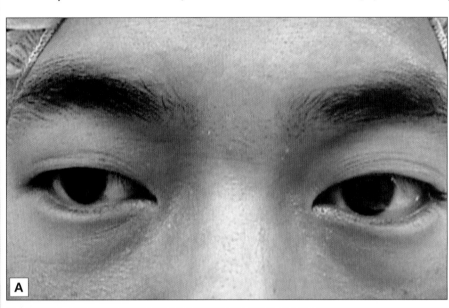

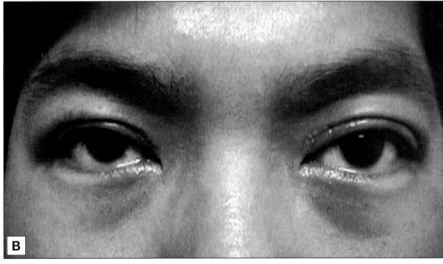

Case 50 (Fig. 14-50 A, B)

31F, absent crease, 5′2″. Prefers average height NTC. I/O: tarsus 7.5 mm. Designed 7.5 mm NTC + 2 mm skin. Observed inferiorly migrated preaponeurotic fat that was bound down. Released and repositioned into superior sulcus. Excised M/C strip. Formed crease.

(B) One week postoperative appearance.

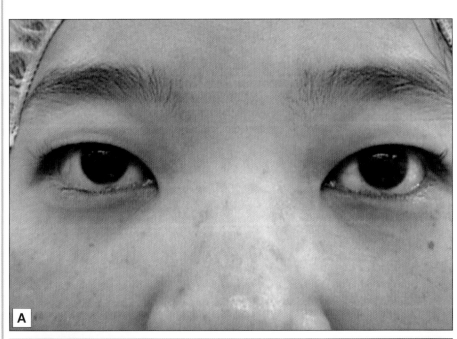

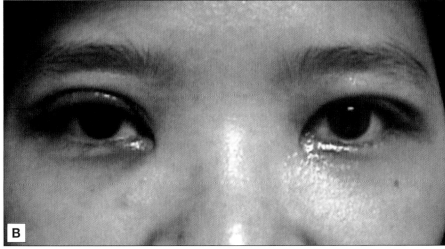

Suboptimal Results and Revision Operations

William P.D. Chen

This chapter shows a variety of cases illustrating suboptimal results of blepharoplasty surgery, and some methods of correction. The contrast between Asian eyelids and those of Caucasians, and the diversity even among Asians themselves, are what makes Asian eyelid surgery a very interesting and challenging art.

Case 1 (Fig. 15-1 A, B)

This patient underwent a lid crease procedure. Notice that the crease does not merge into the fold medially. The medial aspect of the crease overrides the supracanthal fold, resulting in an upper bifid crease.

(B) Higher magnification of RUL.

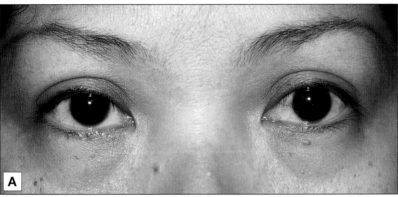

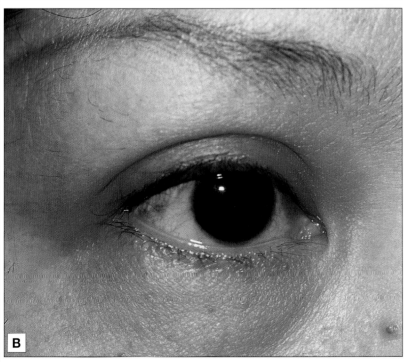

Case 2 (Fig. 15-2 A, B)

A 50-year-old woman with a left seventh nerve palsy who underwent a lid crease procedure. Note the poor closure of her left upper lid owing to facial paresis and probable mid-lamellar contracture.

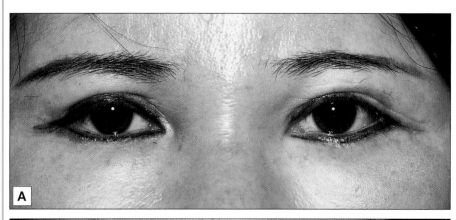

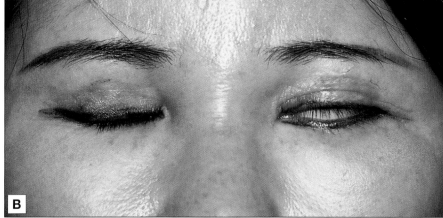

Case 3 (Fig. 15-3)

A 35-year-old woman who has had excessive fat removal high over her supratarsal sulcus. Note the inadequate formation of the lid crease and the hollow sulcus.

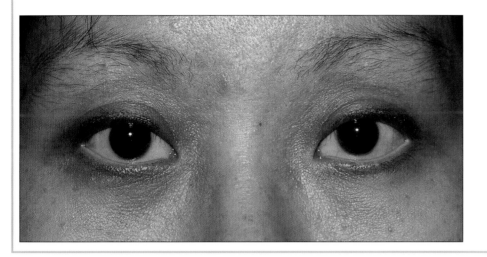

Case 4 (Fig. 15-4 A–C)

Female university student who presented after lid crease placement. (**A**) She showed a high crease over the left upper lid and a segmented crease over the medial extent of the right upper lid and scar over the lateral half of the crease. I recommended enhancement and revision of the right upper crease, and repositioning to a lower level for the left upper crease. She elected to have only the right lid revised. A tarsal height-based Asian blepharoplasty was performed on the right upper lid, cicatrix was released from the lateral half (**B**).

(**C**) One week postoperative appearance.

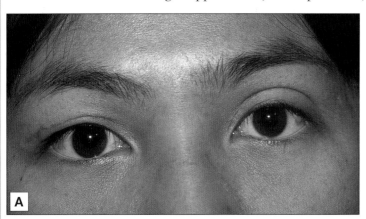

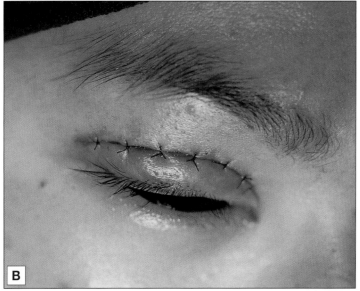

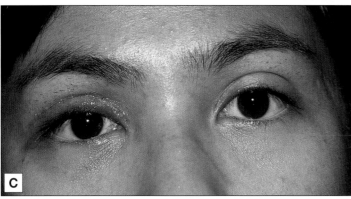

Case 5 (Fig. 15-5)

Incomplete and 'bifid' crease: the upper crease did not extend to the medial one-third of the fissure width. The splitting of the crease is more noticeable over the right upper lid.

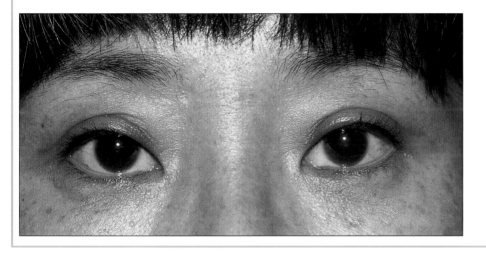

Case 6 (Fig. 15-6 A, B)

A patient with asymmetric creases. The right upper lid crease was too close to the lid margin, and is scarred down to the anterior surface of the upper tarsus. Left upper lid crease is high, harsh, and semilunar in shape.

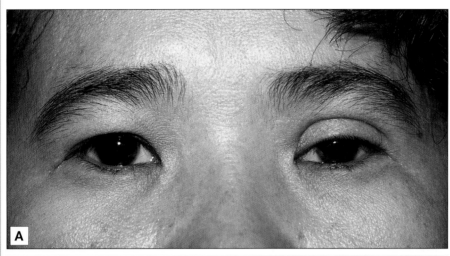

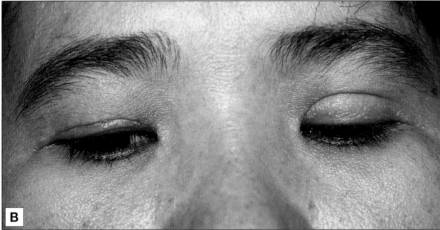

Case 7 (Fig. 15-7 A, B)

A patient had an asymmetric crease made more evident by the acquired ptosis of the right upper lid. This is an example of a static crease.

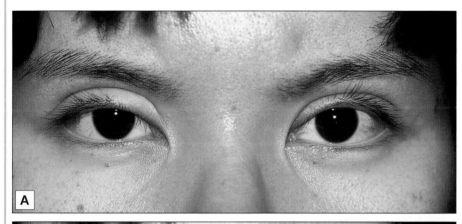

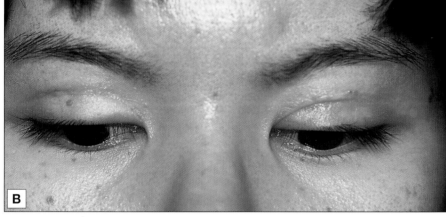

Case 8 (Fig. 15-8 A–C)

(A) A 30-year-old woman with multiple creases over the right upper lid (with one dominant and several less distinct creases over the medial half), and multiple indistinct high creases over the left upper lid. (B) Note the enhanced supratarsal sulcus on the left upper lid, probably due to excessive fat removal. (C) Correction of the left upper lid consisted of crease enhancement with excision of the small strip of skin encompassing the multiple creases. No attempts were made to correct the supratarsal hollow because (a) this is a difficult procedure to perform, and placement of synthetic fillers frequently leads to complications; and (b) the conversion of several faint lines to a main crease often creates enough inward folding, especially on upgaze, to make the hollow less noticeable.

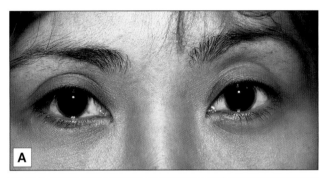

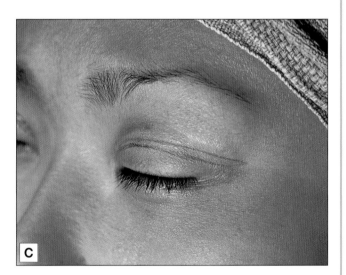

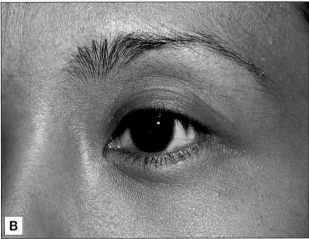

Case 9 (Fig. 15-9)

A 50-year-old woman with high creases, some of which are bifid and multiple.

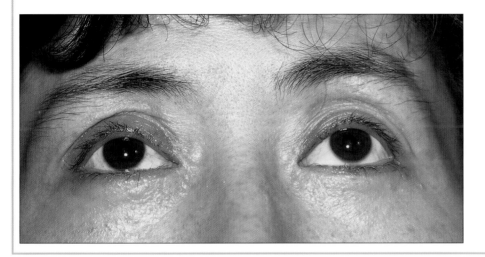

Case 10 (Fig. 15-10 A–D)

(**A**) A 30-year-old woman who had had two lid crease procedures in Asia. She complained that the crease tapered excessively towards the lateral canthi and of fullness in that area when she smiled. (**B**) Asian blepharoplasty was performed laterally. Intraoperatively, scar tissues were excised until the underlying aponeurosis was clearly seen.

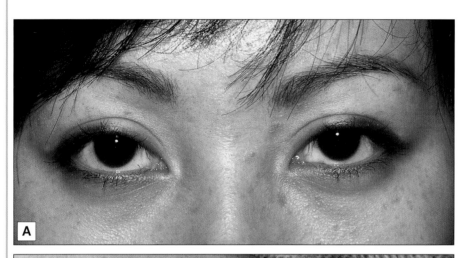

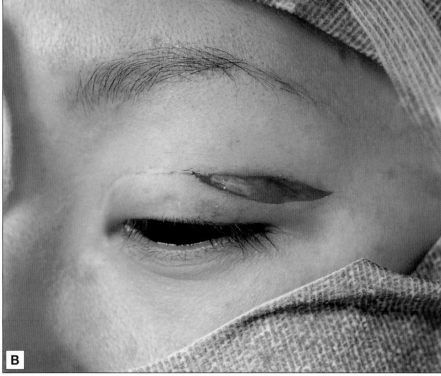

Case 10 (Fig. 15-10 A–D)—cont'd

(C) Appearance immediately after the procedure.
(D) Appearance 1 month postoperatively. Some residual pretarsal edema can still be seen.

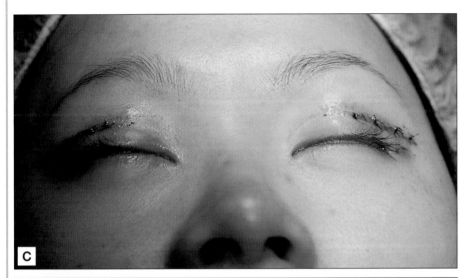

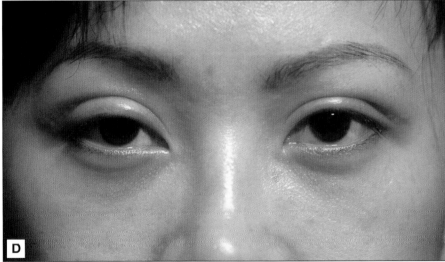

Case 11 (Fig. 15-11 A–E)

(A, B) A 25-year-old patient had undergone place-ment of a reddish tattoo line in an attempt to form a pseudo-crease over the right upper lid. She had mini-mal ptosis of the same lid.

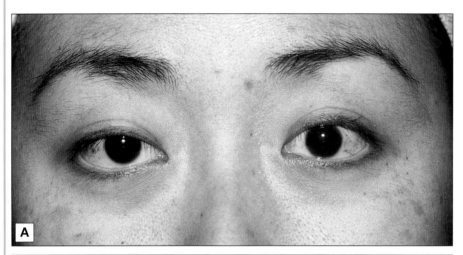

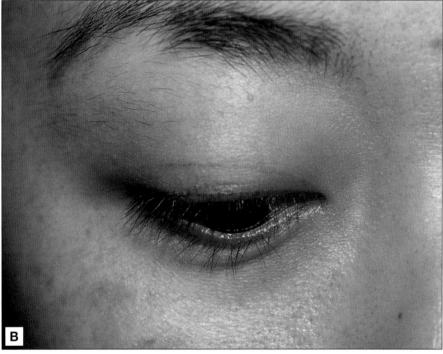

Case 11 (Fig. 15-11 A–E)—cont'd

(**C**) The tattooed crease line, which measured less than 1 mm wide, was excised. (**D**) A new crease was formed based on my technique.

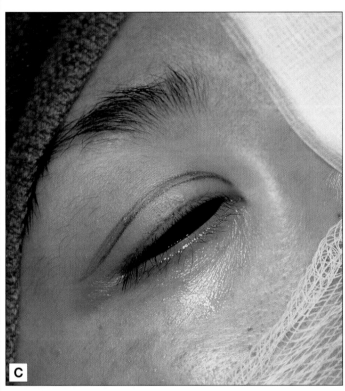

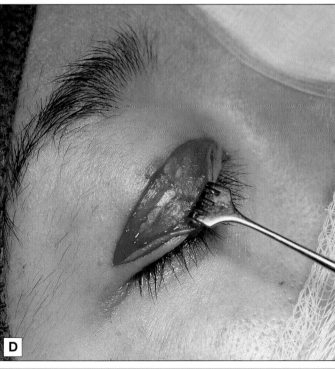

Case 11 (Fig. 15-11 A–E)—cont'd

(E) Closure of wound over right upper lid.

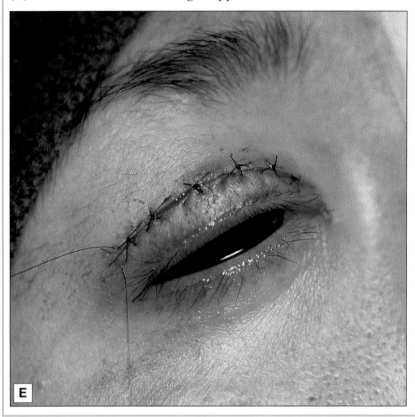

Case 12 (Fig. 15-12)

A 55-year-old woman with a high, harsh, incomplete crease. The crease spanned only 60% of the width of the fissure.

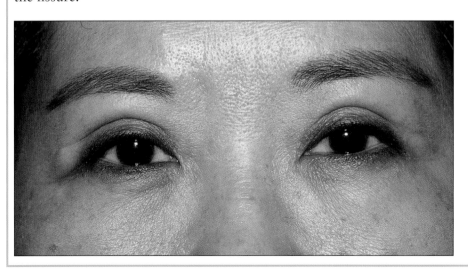

Case 13 (Fig. 15-13 A–C)

(**A**) This patient had a crease deformity of the right upper lid due to laceration by broken windshield glass during an automobile accident with embedded glass fragments. The left upper lid had a 'shielded' crease. (**B, C**) Postoperative views after crease revision.

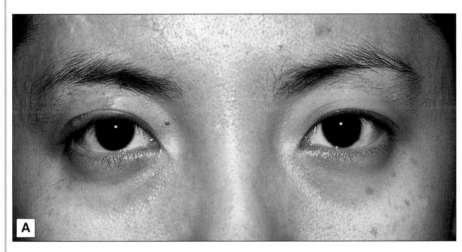

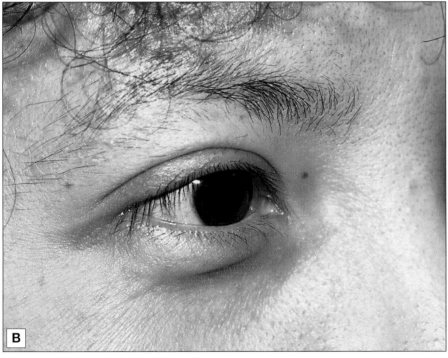

Case 13 (Fig. 15-13 A–C)—cont'd

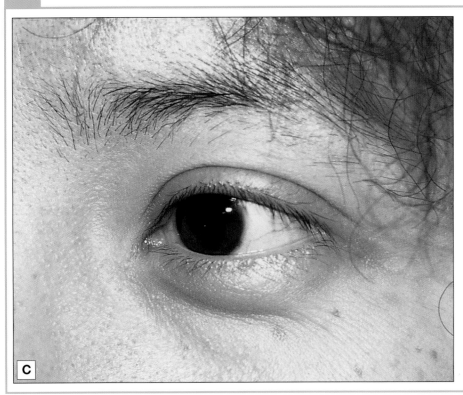

C

Case 14 (Fig. 15-14 A–D)

(**A**) A 28-year-old patient before Asian blepharoplasty.
(**B**) Immediately after the procedure.

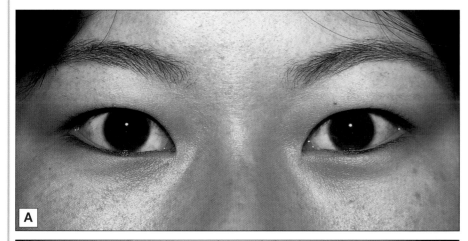

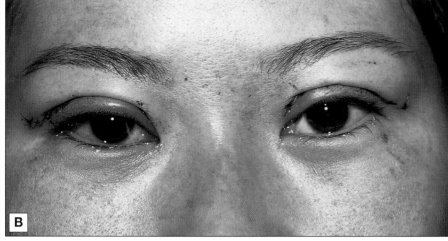

Case 14 (Fig. 15-14 A–D)—cont'd

(C) Six months after the operation the patient reported a 30% weight gain (from 90 to 120 lb) and obliteration of the left upper lid crease. (D) Surgical exploration showed hypertrophy of the suborbicularis (preseptal) fat pads, which may have obliterated previous crease-forming attachment.

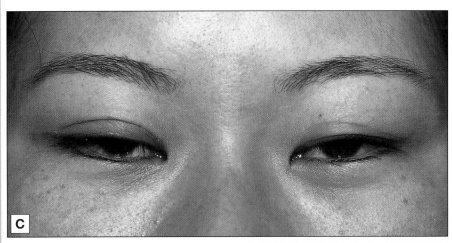

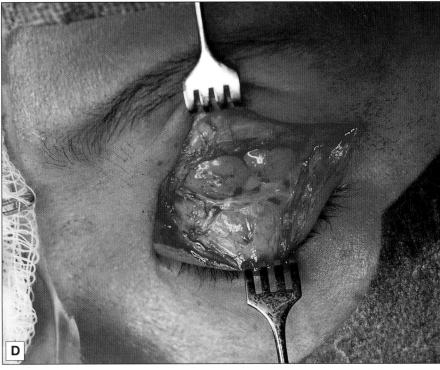

Case 15 (Fig. 15-15 A–I)

(**A**) A 19-year-old woman with absence of lid crease. (**B**) Design of a nasally tapered crease over the right upper lid. (**C**) Opening of the orbital septum and excision of some preaponeurotic fat pads. (**D**) Eyelid before surgical closure.

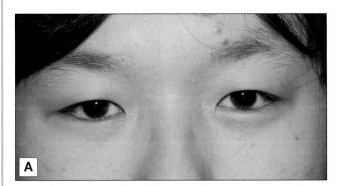

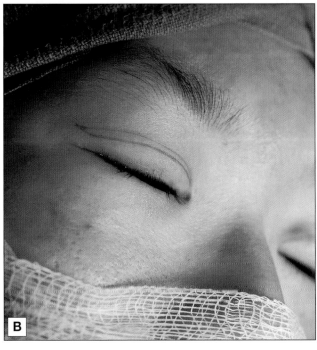

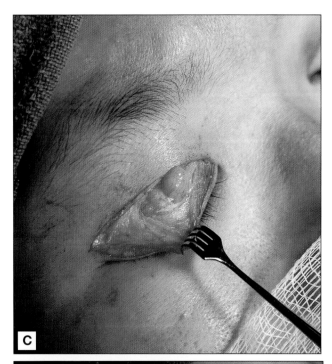

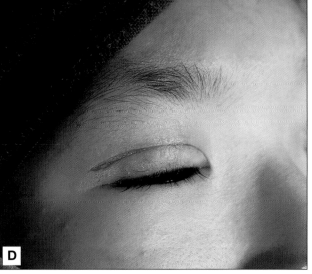

Case 15 (Fig. 15-15 A–I)—cont'd

(E) Closure with both interrupted and continuous 6/0 nylon. (F) Three months postoperatively the crease appeared shallow over the right upper lid, and was incomplete over the lateral portion of the left upper lid. Retrospectively, the patient informed me that because of her anxiety and intolerance to pain she never looked up during the first week after the surgery 'for fear of scarring'. It is most likely that the surgical adhesions did not form adequately during the first week, as the levator muscle was not actively contracted in any way. (G) I performed a revisional Asian blepharoplasty over the right upper lid.

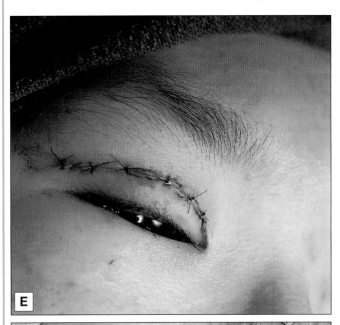

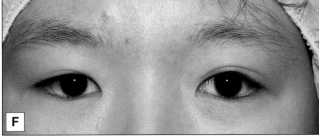

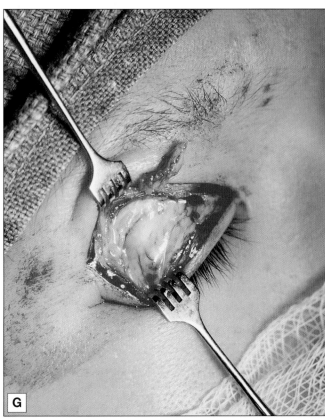

Case 15 (Fig. 15-15 A–I)—cont'd

(H) Enhancement was performed segmentally over the lateral one-third of the left upper lid. **(I)** Appearance immediately after the operation.

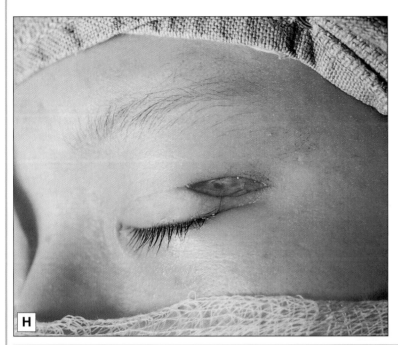

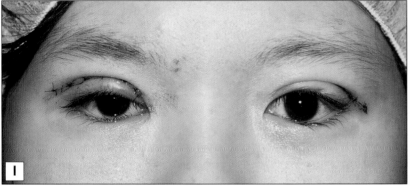

Case 16 (Fig. 15-16 A–E)

(**A**) A 50-year-old woman had previously undergone blepharoplasty and presented with a high parallel crease and some residual hooding of the upper lids. (**B**) Upper and lower lines of incision during revision, the design of the crease allowed for excision of the area of the previous crease incision (dotted line outlined with methylene blue ink) to remove some redundant skin and reposition the crease closer to the lid margin, based on the tarsal height.

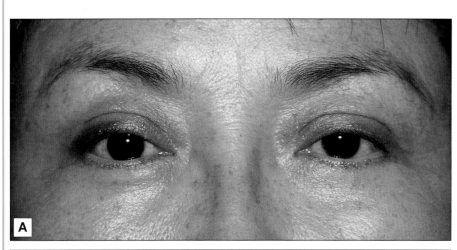

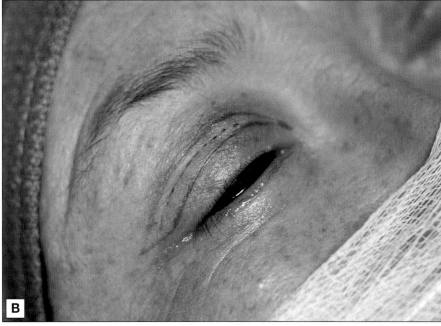

Case 16 (Fig. 15-16 A–E)—cont'd

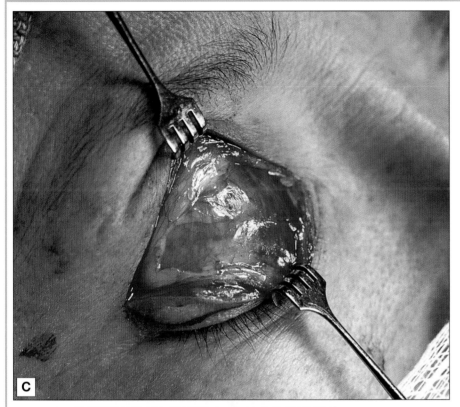

(C) The orbital septum was opened superiorly, revealing minimal preaponeurotic fat pads, which I did not remove. (D) Excision of skin and redundant underlying preseptal orbicularis muscles. The methylene blue tip points to a previously buried 6/0 Prolene suture that had functioned as a levator aponeurosis–inferior subcutaneous fixation suture. (E) Closure of wound following revision.

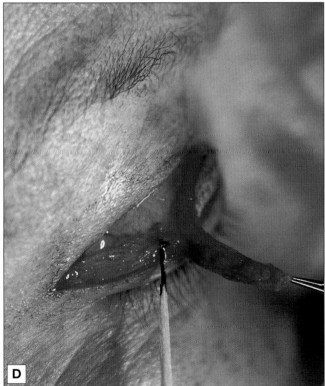

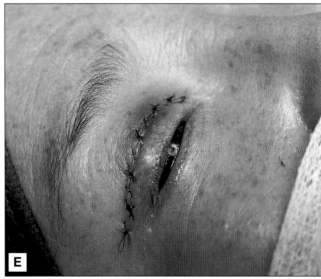

Case 17 (Fig. 15-17 A–D)

(A) A 35-year-old man had seen another surgeon for placement of a lid crease. He later wanted the crease removed or lightened. (B) The creases and the underlying scar tissues on both lids were removed. A persistent crease remained over the lateral half of the right upper lid; the left lid appeared satisfactory. A second procedure was carried out 6 months later to release the subdermal aponeurotic attachment. This resulted in minimal improvement.

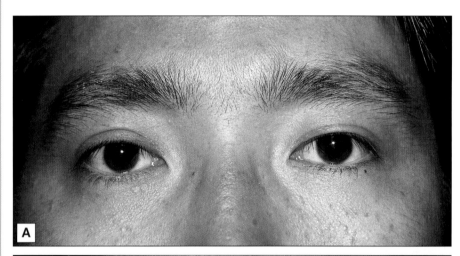

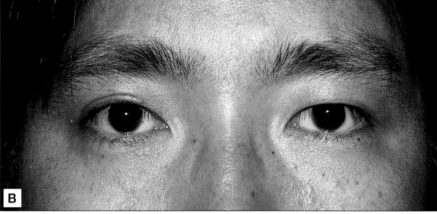

Case 17 (Fig. 15-17 A–D)

(C, D) A year later, I performed a recession of the right upper lid coupled with placement of autolo-gous temporalis fascia. Although the crease faded on downgaze, it could be seen on forward and upgaze.

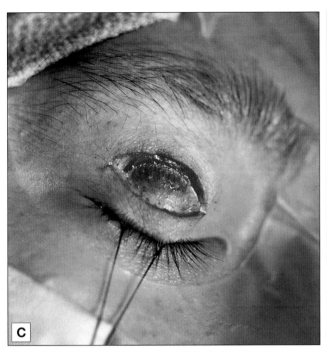

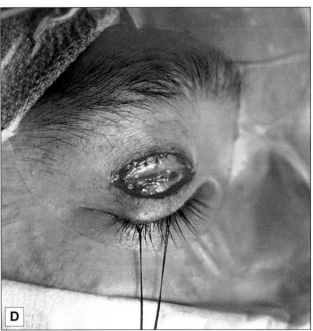

Case 18 (Fig. 15-18 A, B)

23F, 5 years s/p previous crease procedure by me. Crease has disappeared. Her height is 5′5″. Mild degree of fat persisted, with small left medial canthal web (**A**).

I/O: tarsus only 6.5 mm. I used 7 mm to design NTC. Very soft fluctuant pretarsal and preseptal tissues. Lyzed along superior edge's cicatrix and orbicularis. Had amorphous inferiorly migrated fibromosaic fat (preseptal fat) which is then repositioned superiorly. Excised scar and myocutaneous strip.

(**B**) Postoperative appearance.

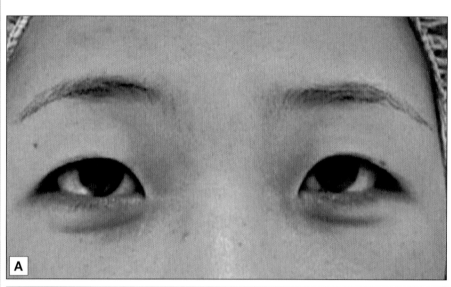

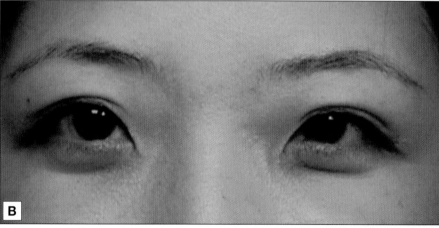

Case 19 (Fig. 15-19 A, B)

46M 2 yrs s/p removal of upper lid hooding. Has rudimentary crease, low-set and dark incisional line with spreading; 3 mm cornea covered (ptosis). Medial incision line measures only 3 mm from lashes. (A&B) Preoperative appearance.

I/O: designed a single 5 mm parallel incisional line as there was no skin redundancy. Lyzed along upper edge of incision until large amount of preseptal and preaponeurotic (postseptal) fat was seen. Debulked scar along the superior tarsal border such that a new crease could form along there.

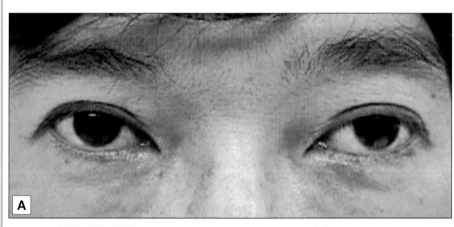

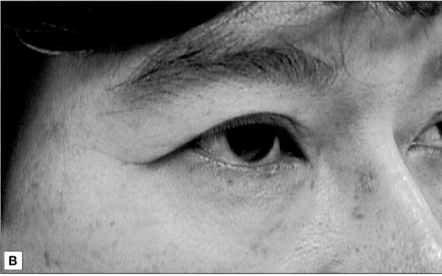

Case 20 (Fig. 15-20 A, B)

27M, 6 yrs s/p lid crease procedure, has high crease and pretarsal fullness. NTC. Right crease height is 9 mm, left is 11–12 mm. Patient feels irritation of the eyelid when blinking (**A**).

I/O: tarsus 6 mm. Past history of ptosis and repair? In this revisional attempt for the LUL, 8.5 mm was chosen to mark an NTC and included 2.5 mm as the amount of skin and scar to be excised. Lyzed along the upper incisional edge to reach the preaponeurotic space. Found and removed two buried stitches. Then excised myocutaneous strip of skin and scar. Reconstructed a shallower NTC.

(**B**) Appearance at two months postoperative. Patient reported a greater degree of comfort when he blinks.

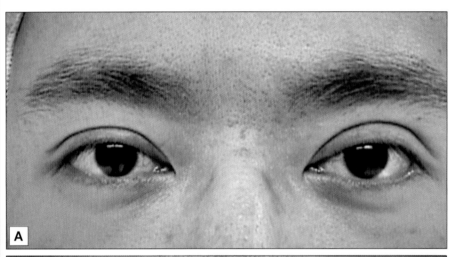

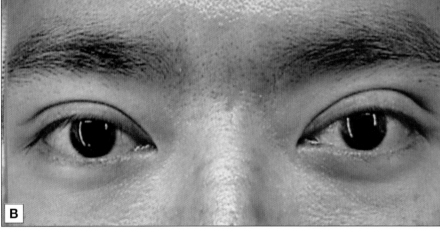

Case 21 (Fig. 15-21)

30F with obliterated crease. Had surgery 6 yrs ago with incisional approach; uses tape for OU daily. Has rudimentary crease RUL, LUL has pigmented incisional spots along medial end of eyelid.

I/O: tarsus 8 mm. Designed 7.5 mm NTC with 1 mm skin, such that the lower incision line was below her previous scar, and included 1 mm of scarred skin only.

RUL; beveled approach along the upper edge to reach the preaponeurotic fat within the remnants of the preaponeurotic space. Although I initially reduced the abundant fat partially with bipolar cautery, the crease did not form well owing to its location along the STB. I reopened the wound and excised the preaponeurotic fat that was along the STB, leaving the upper half mostly intact. It was only then that the crease formed well. Three buried nylon stitches were removed.

LUL also included scar excision. Again excised preaponeurotic fat. The central crease fixation suture did not perform well and was removed; more of the inferior edge tissues were cleared and excised; the 6/0 suture then fixed well, with better crease formation.

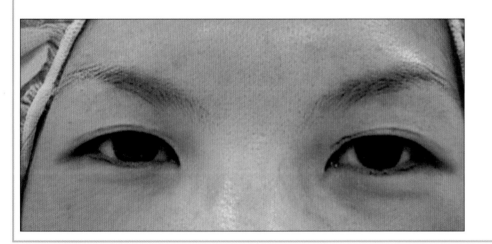

Case 22 (Fig. 15-22 A, B)

20F 4 yrs s/p surgery elsewhere using two-stitch technique from conjunctival side. Has rudimentary crease line. Small fissures with horizontal palpebral width ~0.75". 4+ brow action, 3 mm ptosis. Wanted NTC (A).

I/O: tarsus 8 mm. Designed 7 mm NTC + 2 mm skin. Found large infiltrate of fibrous preseptal fat that appeared to have migrated inferiorly, as well as preaponeurotic fat; both were partially reduced through excision. She had limited upgaze and therefore crease construction relied exclusively on interrupted sutures.

(B) Two months postoperatively.

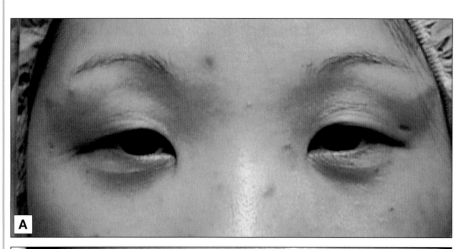

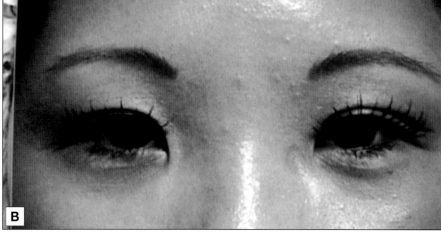

Case 23 (Fig. 15-23)

37M, 12 yrs s/p upper blepharoplasty, with first revision done same year to enhance crease. RUL had been revised by me and was satisfactory. Now desires revision of LUL. LUL has segmentation of medial one-third of crease, with peaking there. Crease measured 8.5 mm and chronic edema had caused an extra fold of skin to appear, as if hanging over the lateral portion of the crease.

I/O: scar at ~8.5 mm. I used 7 mm to design an NTC, encompassing his scar in the 1.5 mm of skin-scar tissues. Used superior beveled approach for this revision to reach the preaponeurotic space. Removed three buried nylon stitches. His voluntary upgaze then showed good crease formation.

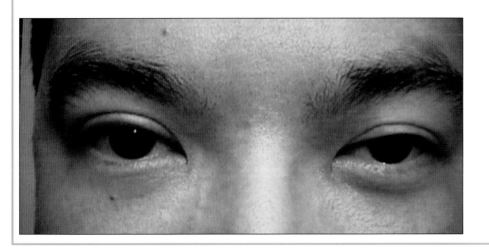

Case 24 (Fig. 15-24 A, B)

21M left eye with congenital ptosis and had levator resection 2 years ago. Six months s/p suture technique O.U. to form crease. RUL medial end has tapered crease, absent crease over LUL. Left upper lid's incision line is only 2–3 mm from lid margin. Feels as if LUL has resistance and discomfort (**A**).

I/O: tarsus 8 mm. Designed incision at 7 mm + 1 mm skin. Removed buried 4/0 Mersilene stitch centrally above STB. Used beveled approach to reach preaponeurotic space. Little fat remains. Excised M/C strip. Used cutting cautery to clear a small trough along anterior tarsal surface just inferior to STB. Used crease fixation sutures from skin to tarsus/aponeurosis and skin.

(**B**) Appearance two months postoperatively.

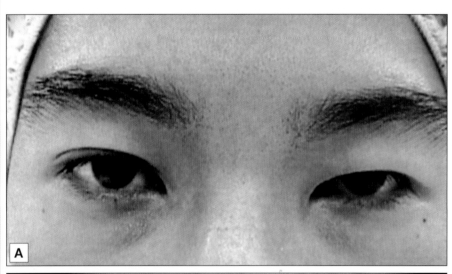

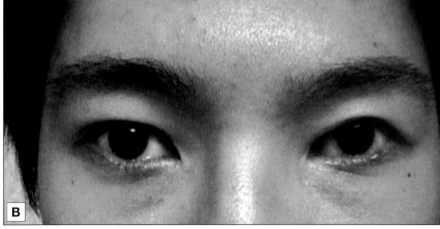

Case 25 (Fig. 15-25 A, B)

42F had upper lid surgery at 27 y/o. Has very high 11–12 mm parallel crease OU. Has slight ptosis, with 2 mm cornea covered OU (**A**).

I/O: tarsus 6.5 mm only. Patient had heavily tattooed permanent eyeliner, which measured 2.5 mm in width from the ciliary margin. Designed crease at 6.5 mm from the upper edge of this permanent eyeliner, therefore at about 9 mm from ciliary margin, as she did not have any residual skin for an ideal revision. Lyzed adhesion through superior incision edge. Released traction and freed up the levator ('up-release') from anterior skin/orbicularis layer; upgaze appeared unrestricted on the operating table. Preaponeurotic fat OU was left untouched. Excised superficial skin scar, 2 mm strip only; avoided injury levator as patient has mild ptosis. Reformed crease. The pretarsal skin has been freed from its attachment to the anchor point of the previously high crease, therefore it has been 'down-released.' When the crease is thus reconstructed, it looks better than the 9 mm that was planned and actually measured at about 7.5 mm from the lid margin, or 5 mm from the upper edge of the permanent eyeliner's border. It has therefore appeared to migrate from an incisional distance of 6.5 mm from the permanent eyeliner to now being at 5 mm from the same margin.

(**B**) Appearance at one week following revision. Patient subsequently informed us that she underwent a brow lift elsewhere at day 4 following our procedure for her.

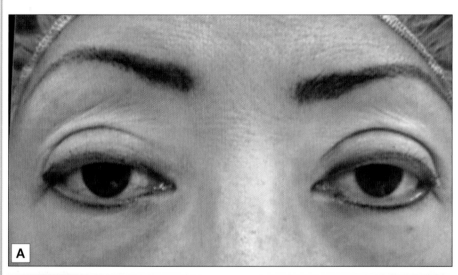

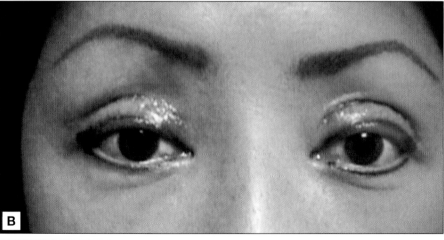

Case 26 (Fig. 15-26 A, B)

60F, 2 years s/p revisional upper blepharoplasty where injection of abdominal free fat graft to upper lid sulcus was performed. Now has prominent hypertrophied and permanent rubbery fat over sulcus and along the superior orbital rim of LUL > RUL, and multiple folds and significant asymmetry (**A**).

I/O: tarsus 6 mm only. Designed crease with 2 mm skin included for excision. Beveled approach to lyze skin adhesion along upper edge of incision first, then secondly through orbicularis/orbital septum complex to reach preaponeurotic space. Observed yellow preaponeurotic fat. Superior to this was consolidated and indurated pale-yellow fat located over the sulcus and anteriorly along the superior orbital rim. Over the LUL a 10 × 30 mm roll of indurated fat graft was excised. Excised M/C strip. Closed wound with 6/0 and 7/0 sutures.

RUL: did not remove fat. Just excised 2 mm skin to revise the crease.

(**B**) Appearance at one week postoperative visit.

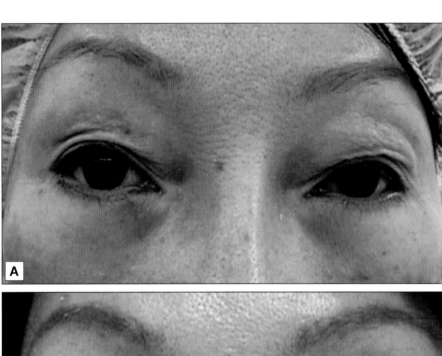

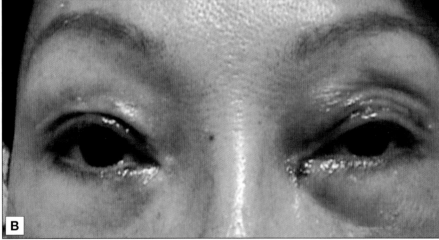

Case 27 (Fig. 15-27)

66F 5 years s/p upper and lower blepharoplasty. Complains of incisional scar over lateral portion of LUL incision that arches towards the lateral canthal angle. Has prominent sulcus.

I/O: beveled approach along upper edge of incision, which was over lateral half of lid only. Levator aponeurosis appears infiltrated by fat; excised 4mm of M/C strip. Reformed crease with greater separation from her lateral canthus.

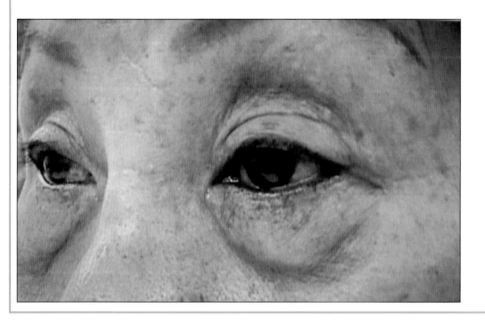

Case 28 (Fig. 15-28 A, B)

30F s/p upper and lower blepharoplasty. Upper crease incisional scar is high and has spread (with right higher than left), with medial angulation over LUL; lower lid subciliary incision line too far from lid margin. Desires revision of upper crease OU and lateral portion of LLL incision line. (A&B) Both pre-revisional appearance.

I/O: tarsus 7 mm. Designed 7 mm crease + 1 mm skin/scar tissue medially, and 2 mm skin/scar laterally.

RUL: beveled approach along upper edge, pre-served orbicularis. Made mini-trough along STB. Applied three 6/0 Vicryl sutures from inferior orbicularis to levator aponeurosis, plus the usual 6/0 interrupted skin/levator/skin sutures as well as 7/0 running suture for skin to skin.

LUL: used only 6/0 interrupted as well as 7/0 running in the usual approach.

LLL: infraciliary approach, excised scar. Tightened inferior limb of lateral canthal ligament by plicating it with 6/0 Vicryl suture.

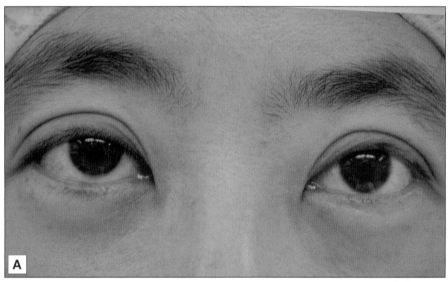

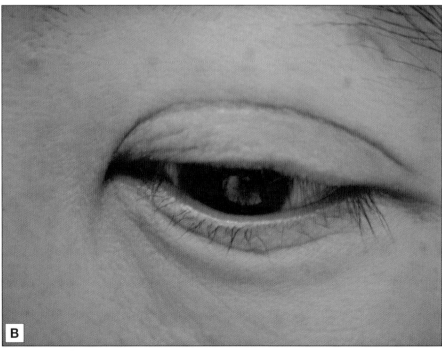

Case 29 (Fig. 15-29 A, B)

Female patient had surgery 4 years ago and a second time a year prior to being seen.

Right upper lid – deep NTC crease, converging, with 3 mm ptosis.

Left upper lid – medial bifurcation of crease as it approaches the medial canthal fold.

Levator function R 12 mm, L 15 mm. Appears esotropic. Height 5′0″.

I/O: RUL harsh and static 12 mm crease, bound down. Tarsus measured 6 mm. Designed 6 mm NTC.

Incision with no. 15 blade, then used blunt-tipped Westcott spring scissors to lyze adhesions along superior edge until preaponeurotic fat is seen (no true septum left). Used cutting cautery to remove scar and redundancy along preaponeurotic platform, plus removal of 8/0 nylon buried sutures that were used for crease formation. Formed crease with 6/0 and 7/0 silk sutures that were removed after 5 days.

(A&B) Both are pre-revisional appearance.

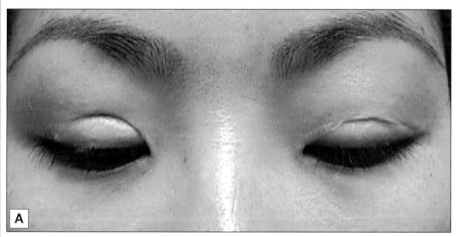

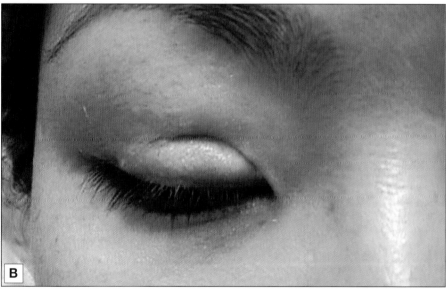

Case 30 (Fig. 15-30)

Female patient underwent lid crease procedure 7 years ago. RUL hooded and rudimentary crease. LUL has high crease with bifid ending both corners.

I/O: tarsus measured 7 mm. Designed NTC OU.

RUL: removed 2 mm skin and orbicularis. Used scissors to go through upper edge of incision, staying beveled to reach preaponeurotic plane.

LUL: eliminated bifid crease, removed buried nylon sutures.

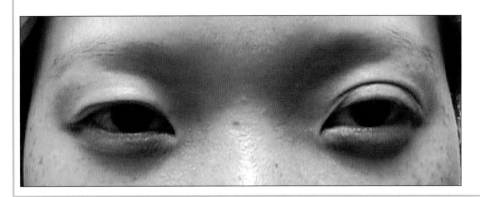

Case 31 (Fig. 15-31)

47 y/o female patient with first surgery 20 years ago coupled with 'W-plasty.' Then revision 12 years ago.

I/O: observed prominent medial pre-aponeurotic fat as well as nasal fat pad. Removed fat pads. Use

6/0 Vicryl to fixate inferior orbicularis to levator and then superior edge of orbicularis; kept suture knot buried.

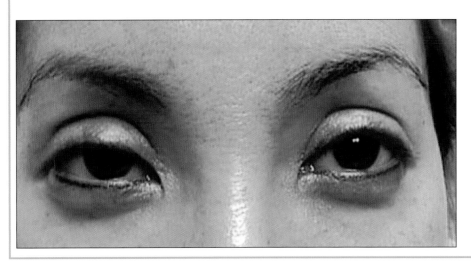

Case 32 (Fig. 15-32)

29 y/o housewife. Had surgery at 18 in Korea. Crease appears high OU. RUL appears deep-set. Has moderate fullness over pretarsal area. LUL is more converged medially than that of the RUL.

I/O: tarsus was only 5.5–6 mm. RUL crease measured 11 mm, LUL at 10 mm. Designed 8.5 mm parallel crease over RUL with some tapering medially; and 8 mm over LUL in an attempt to equalize two asymmetric high creases. Use blunt scissors to reach preaponeurotic space superiorly. Large amount of cicatrix over preseptal as well as pretarsal zones. Excised strip of myocutaneous flap OU. Excised strip of pretarsal inferior orbicularis muscle to reduce fullness. Checked levator's excursion on the table and appeared normal OU.

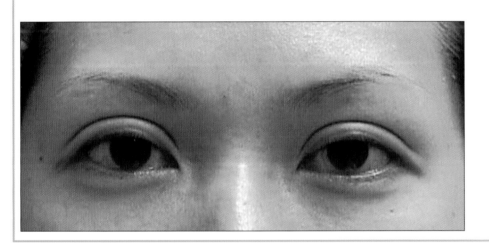

Case 33 (Fig. 15-33)

55 y/o had four-lid blepharoplasty 10 years previously in Hawaii. Has high bifid semilunar creases OU, measured to be 10–11 mm in sulcus.

I/O: designed parallel crease OU at 7.5 mm (tarsus measured 7 mm). Excised old crease with 1 mm clear skin superior to it, with the lower skin incision edge at 7.5 mm. Found very attenuated levator muscle with fatty infiltration. Formed parallel crease.

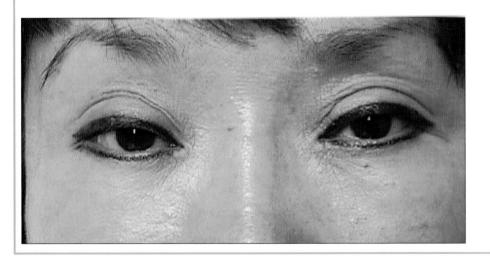

Case 34 (Fig. 15-34)

29 y/o had crease procedure 9 years earlier: stitch method alone, with adjustment attempted twice. LUL has no crease. RUL has shallow NTC. Patient prefers parallel crease.

I/O: very vascular. Removed buried nylon sutures from along the superior tarsal border. Used 6/0 silk and 6/0 Prolene with significant attachment towards the levator aponeurosis.

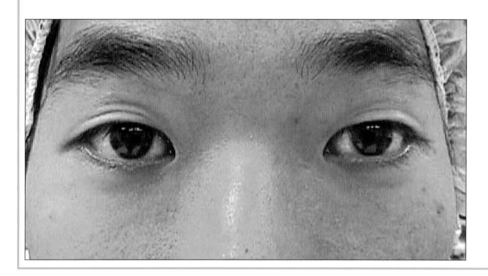

Case 35 (Fig. 15-35)

36 y/o 3 years status post lid crease procedure. Currently has shielded crease over RUL, and LUL has wider separation from lid margin than the RUL. Wants parallel crease.

I/O: designed 7 mm crease height to encompass RUL scar. Excised moderate amount of preaponeurotic fat from RUL as well as inferior orbicularis strip.

LUL: reduced the crease height medially. Fat not as excessive and therefore only reduced some with bipolar Wetfield cautery. Excised inferior orbicularis strip. Closed with 6/0 silk. Inspection revealed this LUL crease still high. Take down and re-excise small amount of skin from lower edge. Result was more symmetrical look.

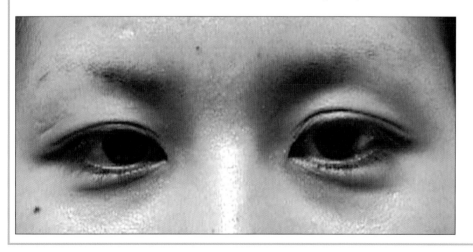

Case 36 (Fig. 15-36)

24 y/o had lid crease procedure in Hong Kong 8 years previously. RUL crease never formed and is now shallow; LUL crease is deeper, but central portion slightly peaked. Desired NTC.

I/O: RUL tarsus measures 6.5 mm. Used 7 mm to design an NTC. Resected scar tissue, no fat. Used 6/0 and 7/0 silk.

LUL: 'square-well' excision of strip of scar tissue along superior tarsal border. Mid-section underwent some dissection superiorly to release fibrosis down to the aponeurosis. Reformed smooth NTC, with good result.

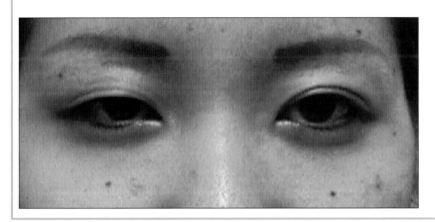

Case 37 (Fig. 15-37)

Male patient, 9 years previously had lid crease procedure. The crease did not fold in well by the end of the first week. Revised 2 months later, with same finding. Has very faint rudimentary line OU. Patient wanted the medial one-third of the crease to be lifted higher. However, this would lead to a triangular or rectangular look. After careful discussion, the patient chose a parallel crease.

I/O: tarsus measured 8 mm. We designed a 7 mm parallel crease. Lyzed scar tissues along the upper incisional edge, through orbicularis. Observed amor-phous fat plastered against levator muscle. After the skin muscle flap was trimmed, there were still remnants of preseptal tissues along the superior tarsal border; as the patient looks up this redundant tissue would bunch up and make the crease look low and 'rope-like'. This was then excised to show a clean insertion of the aponeurosis along the superior tarsal border. The lower skin edge was pulled up and united with the aponeurosis along the superior tarsal border, forming a nice parallel 7 mm crease.

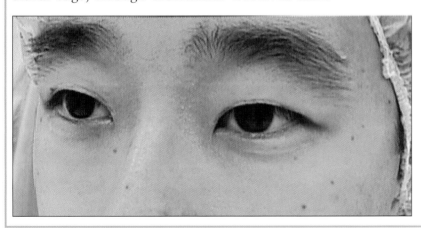

Case 38 (Fig. 15-38)

30 y/o who was 10 years status post external incision crease procedure. The lateral extent of the RUL appears to downslant towards the lateral canthus. The incisional line has spread over the left side. Desires parallel crease to be of above average height.

I/O: tarsus measures 8 mm. Used a parallel 8 mm incision line, included 2.5 mm skin. Very vascular orbicularis oculi muscle. Preaponeurotic fat pad protrudes inferiorly over the lateral half and required partial excision. The rest of the fat seemed spread out and plastered down. Formed crease with 6/0 and 7/0 silk.

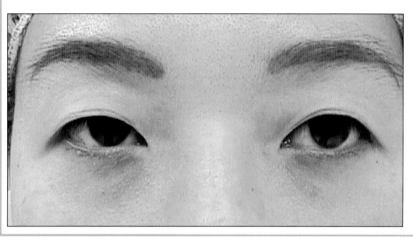

Case 39 (Fig. 15-39)

19 y/o. Heavy upper lid hooding with fat. Some brow action. Wants to have hooding and fat removed but does not want crease formation. Height 5′3″.

I/O: tarsus measured 7 mm. Used hyaluronidase in local injection. Made lower incision line at 5 mm and included 3 mm of skin in a parallel configuration. After using blade through skin, I used cutting cautery with very fine tip to traverse through the upper edge of the orbicularis. Reached septum and opened it. Excised 80% of prolapsing preaponeurotic fat. Excised myocutaneous strip that consisted mostly of skin, leaving behind half of the orbicularis along the superior tarsal border. Closed orbicularis to orbicularis with 6/0 Vicryl. Skin closed with 6/0 nylon in a running fashion, taking bites of skin only. No interrupted sutures were used on the skin.

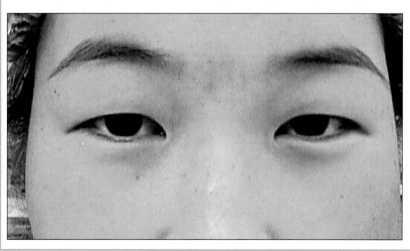

Case 40 (Fig. 15-40 A, B)

22 y/o. Four years status post lid crease procedure and attempted ptosis repair of the right upper lid. RUL crease is deep set and height was 8 mm, with 1.5 mm of cornea covered. LUL has deep-set 6 mm crease, 0.5 mm cornea is covered. (**A&B**) Preoperative appearance.

I/O: measured right tarsus and it was only 5.5 mm, probably had tarsectomy. LUL tarsus measured 7 mm.

RUL very vascular. Created 7 mm NTC and included 2 mm skin. Found three blue nylon stitches, scarred levator/tarsus junction. Performed external resection of 3 mm of aponeurosis. Dissected epitarsally to smooth out already swollen tarsal area. Formed crease with 6/0 and 7/0 silk.

LUL: also set crease height at 7 mm, and NTC. Found three nylon stitches and removed them. Excised 1.5 mm skin–muscle strip. Formed crease.

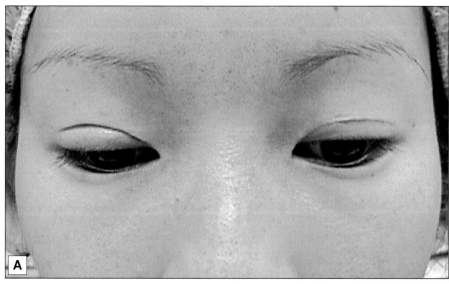

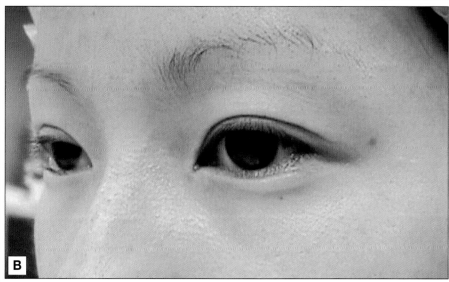

Case 41 (Fig. 15-41 A, B)

36 y/o who was 10 years post first crease procedure.

RUL had 12 mm crease height with broad medial portion;

LUL had 14 mm deep crease. Height is 5'7". (A)

I/O: tarsus measured 7 mm. Used 8 mm as crease. Included 3 mm skin segment. Opened preaponeurot- ic plane with bevelled Westcott scissors along the upper edge. No fat seen. Formed crease with 6/0 and 7/0 silk.

(B) Postoperative appearance at three weeks.

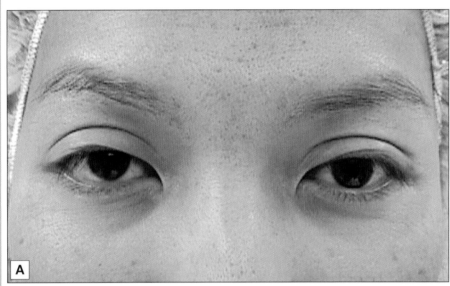

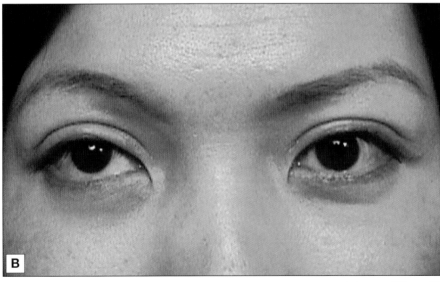

Case 42 (Fig. 15-42)

66 y/o Right upper lid with 3 mm ptosis, hollow sulcus and absent crease. LUL has high crease. Levator function RUL 7 mm, LUL 14 mm.

I/O: RUL has had previous tarsectomy-type procedure. Applied frontal nerve block. Performed lysis of adhesion along the superior edge of the skin incision. Levator was extremely attenuated. The aponeurosis was elevated from underlying conjunctiva and 10 mm was resected. The edge of the muscle was then advanced and reanastomosed inferiorly along the STB using 6/0 Vicryl. Formed crease with multiple 6/0 and 7/0 silk sutures.

LUL: created 6 mm crease line incision, then dissected upwards towards scar to reach preaponeurotic plane. Resected the old cicatrix and fragment of skin between it and the new lower edge of the crease incision.

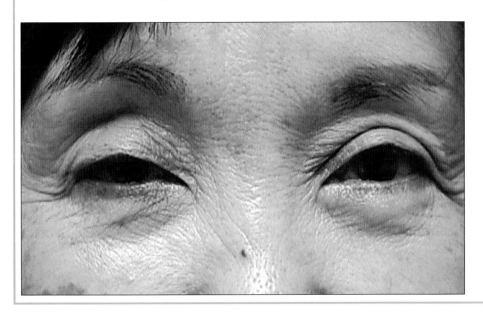

Case 43 (Fig. 15-43)

23 y/o with rudimentary crease OU. The upper lid margin appeared to peak over the medial one-third and gave a triangular look. Desired nasally tapered crease. I performed Asian blepharoplasty. Five years later both sides creases have disappeared. Eyelids now appear just as full, even though first procedure had involved preaponeurotic fat excision.

I/O: tarsus measured 6.5 mm. Used 7 mm to mark crease. Had very soft fluctuant pretarsal and presep-tal tissues. Had amorphous downwardly migrated preseptal (sub-brow) fat which was disrupting the crease formation. This was repositioned superiorly. Excised scar and myocutaneous flap. Formed crease with 6/0 and 7/0 silk in a nasally tapered configuration.

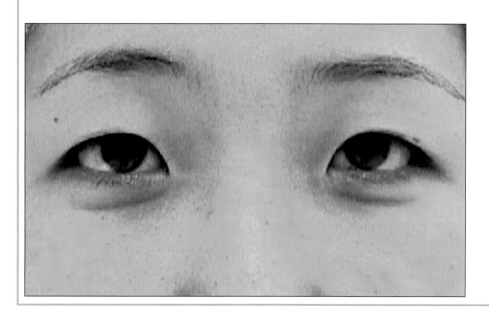

Case 44 (Fig. 15-44 A, B)

23 y/o with small palpebral fissure and mild ptosis OU. (A) Prior to any procedure. (B) One year following Asian Blepharoplasty she developed shallowing of crease over both upper eyelids.

I/O: RUL tarsus measured 6.5 mm. Designed crease including less than 1 mm of previous incision line. Lyzed superior edge of incision through orbicularis. No unusual fat seen. Presence of thick fluctuant preseptal orbicularis was seen; this was excised.

LUL: crease form was borderline after closure. Released the sutures and re-fixated by deeper placement on to aponeurosis. The medial portion of the levator aponeurosis appeared to have some fat infiltration.

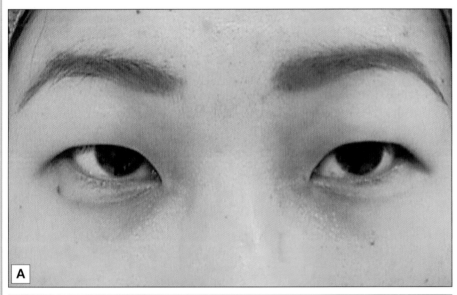

A

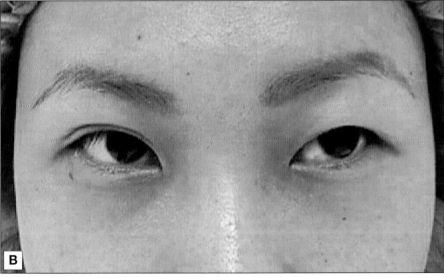

B

The Concept of a Glide Zone as it Relates to Upper Lid Crease, Lid Fold, and its Application in Primary and Revisional Blepharoplasty

Chapter 16

William P.D. Chen

The normal eyelid can be conceptualized as consisting of two main layers anatomically: the anterior skin–orbicularis oculi muscle layer, and the posterior layers of the levator muscle, or levator aponeurosis, Müller's muscle, and adherent conjunctiva.

In general, Caucasian eyelids with a crease are thinner than their Asian counterparts owing to a combination of factors, including a higher point of fusion of the orbital septum on to the levator aponeurosis; the relatively higher position of the preaponeurotic fat pads and the resultant thinner eyelid segment; the greater number of distal fibers of the levator aponeurosis that terminate towards the skin along the superior tarsal border and above it to form the eyelid crease; and the smaller amount of preseptal fat and the thinner orbicularis. When the levator contracts, the tarsal plate vectors upward and the eyelid crease invaginates easily. Non-Asians may often have a deep-set supratarsal sulcus (Fig. 16-1).

Asians eyelids are further broadly divided into two groups, those with an upper lid crease and those without. In Asians with a crease, although the eyelid may still be thicker than in Caucasians, there is still the presence of distal fibers of the levator aponeurosis terminating towards the skin along the superior tarsal border.[1] Despite the low point of fusion of the orbital septum, when the levator contracts there is an invagination of skin along the superior tarsal margin to form a clinically apparent upper eyelid crease.[2] When the eyes are open and the subject is looking ahead, there is a greater degree of fullness in the preseptal region than in a Caucasian with a crease, but less than that typically seen in Asians without an upper lid crease (Fig. 16-2).

Asians who are without a lid crease typically have thicker eyelids owing to the presence of hypertrophied orbicularis as well as preseptal fat in the pretarsal and supratarsal areas. The orbital septum fuses with the levator aponeurosis at a lower point than in Caucasians with an upper lid crease. There are relatively few fibers or no attachment from the levator aponeurosis towards the skin along the superior tarsal border. Both the pretarsal and the preseptal zone are thick compared to Asians or Caucasians with an upper eyelid crease (Fig. 16-3).

In Asian blepharoplasty, where the goal is to create an ethnically appropriate and aesthetic upper eyelid crease for an individual born without one, two main methods are used to achieve this goal. The first method is suture ligation,[3-6] which is often mentioned as being less invasive, simpler to perform, and relying on the use of buried ligatures to tighten the soft tissues over and along the superior tarsal border, including orbicularis, levator aponeurosis, and Müller's muscle. The second major category is the external incisional approach, whereby a skin incision is made along the designed crease and varying amounts of skin, orbicularis oculi, orbital septum, an optional amount of preaponeurotic fat, or combinations of the above may be removed; this is then coupled with various methods of crease construction using fixation or attachment of the skin to the levator aponeurosis, skin to tarsus along the superior tarsal border, or orbicularis to levator aponeurosis.

The surgical results often depend on a complex interaction between the absence or presence of excessive amounts of tissue overlying the pretarsal zone, as well as over the preseptal area (or midzone of the upper eyelid, between the pretarsal area and the brow); whether the amount of fat is abundant; whether the skin is thin or thickened over each of the two zones mentioned above; the position of the globe itself (normal versus relative proptosis or enophthalmos); the position of the brow; the intrinsic ability of the levator muscle to perform its natural function of opening and elevating the upper lid (measured as 'levator function' – the vertical excursion of the upper eyelid, measuring the upper lid margin from a downgaze position to an upgaze position, and usually expressed in millimeters); as well as whether clinically one sees a firm pretarsal complex of skin adherent to orbicularis/tarsus, versus the opposite scenario of a diffuse inferior accumulation

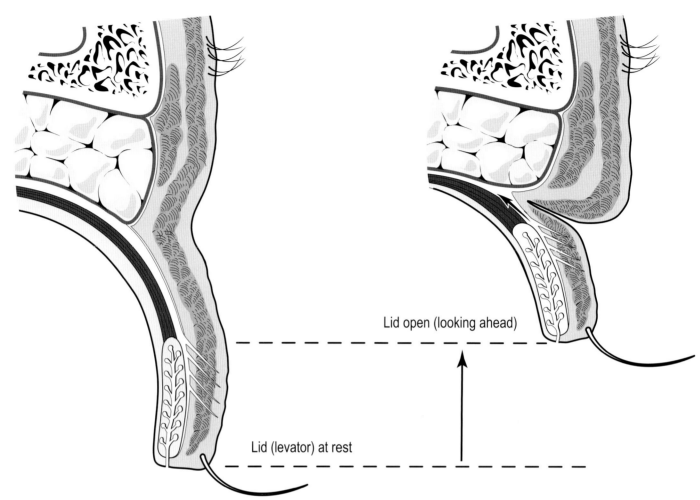

Fig. 16-1 Caucasian eyelid with a crease. In general, Caucasian eyelids with a crease are thinner than their Asian counterparts. This is due to a combination of factors, including a higher point of fusion of the orbital septum on to the levator aponeurosis, the relatively higher position of the preaponeurotic fat pads and the resultant thinner eyelid segment, the greater number of distal fibers of the levator aponeurosis that terminate towards the skin along the superior tarsal border and above to form the eyelid crease, less preseptal fat, and a thinner orbicularis. When the levator contracts, the tarsal plate vectors upward and the eyelid crease invaginates easily.

Within the figure: Lid open (looking ahead); Lid (levator) at rest

of soft tissue over the pretarsal region. In a normal upper eyelid with or without a crease, when the eyes are looking straight ahead and the lids are open, the anterior layer of the skin and orbicularis is in passive relaxation, allowing the posterior layer, consisting of the levator and Müller's muscle, to actively contract and pull the lid margin upward into an open position. The posterior layer of levator–Müller's muscle only has to fold upward and inward for 2–4 mm relative to the anterior layer of skin–orbicularis for a reasonable crease to be observed clinically. The anterior layer of the upper lid therefore offers very little resistance and does not act as a 'resisting platform' against the levator muscle (posterior layer); exceptions to this include heavy eyelids (eyelids with abundant preaponeurotic fat, excessive suborbicularis fat, excessive fat-infiltrated orbicularis, or subcutaneous loose areolar tissues) and poor levator function, including the presence of true ptosis.

The preaponeurotic space and the presence of fat within it is often seen as a hindrance to any attempt at surgical construction of a crease; and the surgical dictum requires that at least a portion of it be excised. There is nothing inherently wrong with this concept; in fact, when the patient presents with excessive soft tissues along the preaponeurotic platform, this author has advocated a beveled approach towards the preaponeurotic space along the upper incision line and,

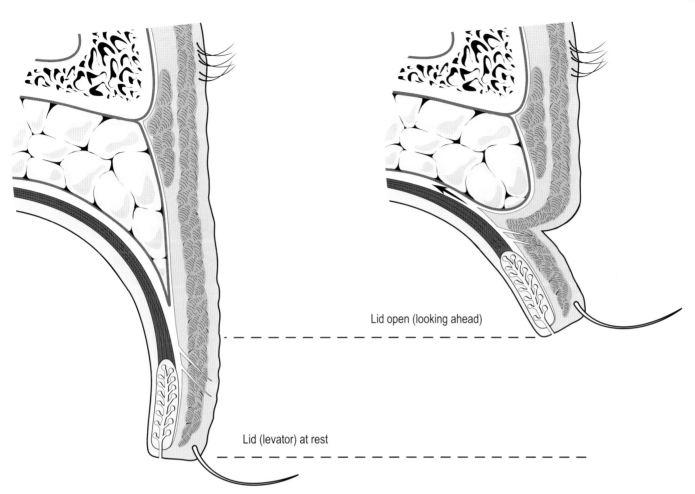

Lid open (looking ahead)

Lid (levator) at rest

Fig. 16-2 Asian with a crease. Although the eyelid may still be thicker than in Caucasians with an upper lid crease, there are distal fibers of the levator aponeurosis terminating towards the skin along the superior tarsal border. Despite the low point of fusion of the orbital septum, when the levator contracts there is an invagination of the skin along the superior tarsal margin to form a clinically apparent upper eyelid crease. When the lids are open and the subject is looking ahead, there is a greater degree of fullness in the preseptal region than in a Caucasian with a crease, but less than that typically seen in Asians without an upper lid crease.

in a clean uniform fashion, performs a uniform trapezoidal debulking of the skin, orbicularis, and small amount of orbital septum, as well as a very small portion of the inferiorly migrated fat.[7] (The fat may be encroaching along the superior tarsal border, the distal portion of the levator aponeurosis over the upper half of the anterior surface of the tarsal plate, as well as its main attachment along the superior tarsal border.) When this is performed prudently and correctly, the presence of fat in the preaponeurotic space is preserved after the crease is constructed. If, after 10 or more years, I should need to re-enter this space using a beveled approach, I can identify the preaponeurotic space and its fat quite readily.

The problem arises when the initial procedure may have involved an overly aggressive excision of the preaponeurotic fat (often the entire portion of the fat in the surgical field), or was accompanied by excessive intra- or postoperative hemorrhage within that space, which is surrounded by orbicularis oculi in front as well as vertical communicating arterial branches of the marginal arcade, the peripheral arcade, and the deep orbital arcade (see discussion in Chapter 2: Vascular Supply of the Upper Eyelid, regarding the arterial distribution of the upper eyelid). The patient often develops a sunken supratarsal sulcus with loss of fullness or contour to the preseptal zone (midzone), and may have poor crease invagination, a seemingly stiffened eyelid

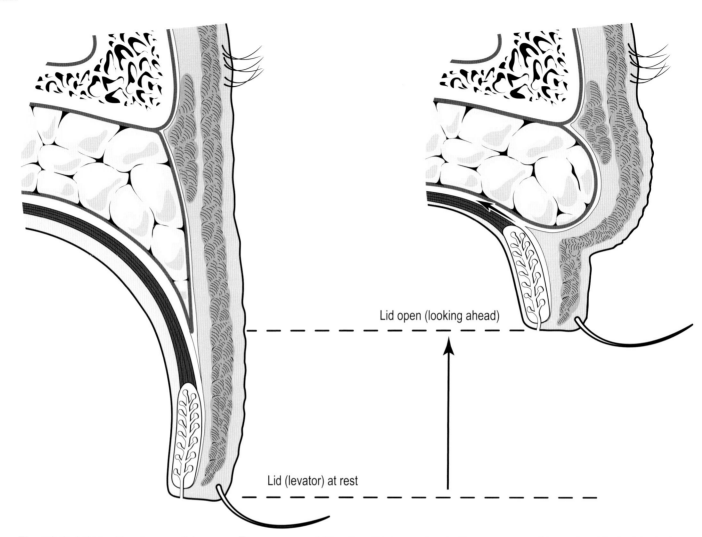

Fig. 16-3 Asian without an eyelid crease. The upper eyelid is often thicker owing to the presence of hypertrophied orbicularis as well as preseptal fat in the pretarsal as well as the supratarsal area. The orbital septum fuses with the levator aponeurosis at a lower point than in Caucasians with an upper eyelid crease. There are relatively few fibers or no attachment from the levator aponeurosis towards the skin along the superior tarsal border. Both the pretarsal and the preseptal zones are thick compared to Asians or Caucasians with an upper eyelid crease.

Lid open (looking ahead)

Lid (levator) at rest

skin, and underlying cicatrix overlying the pretarsal as well as the preseptal area (Fig. 16-4). During revisional surgery one sees a collapse or obliteration of the preaponeurotic space, associated with the absence of preaponeurotic fat. The anterior and the posterior layers appear fused into a single layered complex. The lid crease was not established even in the presence of seemingly adequate levator function. One can visualize this as if the levator muscle now has to carry or lift the pretarsal skin–tarsus complex against the weight of a double load of eyelid layers, as opposed to the usual scenario where the tarsal plate (continuing as the levator layer) glides up and under the anterior layers of

skin and orbicularis muscle. With the anterior layer collapsing on to the posterior layer, the skin–orbicularis is now acting as a 'resisting layer' towards the action of the posterior layer of levator muscle. The absence or presence of this 'glide zone' (with non-adherent preaponeurotic fat within its space) between the two layers can therefore hinder or facilitate the formation of the crease, where a firm tarsal platform is needed to vector upwards against a physiologically and anatomically appropriate amount of preseptal skin and orbicularis oculi. The excursion of this glide or shift of the posterior layer relative to the anterior layer can be a mere 2–4 mm to be effective in manifesting a crease.

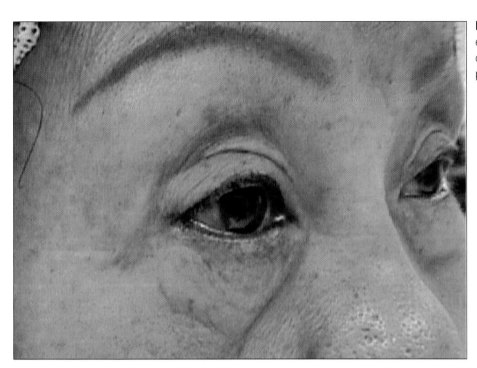

Fig. 16-4 Scarred upper lid. Stiffened eyelid skin with underlying cicatrix overlying the pretarsal as well as the preseptal area.

I have observed the presence of tightly bound preaponeurotic fat in some individuals with a single eyelid presenting for primary surgery; the amorphous infiltrated fat (rather than soft preaponeurotic fat) here in the 'glide zone' may have contributed to the absence of an observable crease in these particular patients. Careful repositioning of this fibrosed fat at a higher level seems to facilitate the up-vectoring of the lid and crease formation.

The properly functioning eyelid crease was described by Boo-Chai[8,9] as being like the visor of a motorcycle helmet; Flowers,[10] in his paper on anchor blepharoplasty, also mentioned the concept that the inferior extent of the preaponeurotic fat acts like a 'ball bearing' at the orbital septum–aponeurotic fusion point (the inferior extent of the preaponeurotic space).

My concept varies from the above in the following way. I see the entire preaponeurotic space – its presence as well as its preservation with some fat within – as a necessary 'third space' or 'third layer'. This middle layer or 'glide zone' includes the preaponeurotic fat and space; it spans the entire width and anterior surface of the levator muscle as well as its aponeurosis, and should be preserved pristinely as much as is feasible (Fig. 16-5). The middle zone (glide zone) where the preaponeurotic fat pads are located is colored yellow and acts as a frictionless lubricating layer which allows the posterior layer to glide upwards. When the patient looks from down to straight ahead with the eyelid open, the levator (agonist) contracts while the sphincter-like pretarsal, preseptal, and periorbital layers of the orbicularis relax. The orbicularis muscle of the upper lid is anchored at the medial and lateral canthal commissures, fusing there as a component of the medial and lateral canthal ligaments. The anterior layer therefore acts like a passive layer, affected by gravity as the posterior layer of the active levator and Müller's muscle contracts to open the eyelid from a closed position. The up-vectoring of the semirigid tarsal plate therefore depends on the middle layer (the glide zone) to allow it to hinge upwards against the passively resisting anterior layer to form an upper lid crease. The anterior layer glides passively over the posterior layer (upper part of the tarsal plate) for several millimeters in the process of forming the upper lid crease; the portion of skin overhanging the tarsal plate is the eyelid fold.

The absence of abnormal adhesion as well as the presence of cushioning fat within this glide zone allows the pretarsal platform to shift and glide slightly posterosuperiorly under the preseptal eyelid to form a physiological upper lid crease. As previously mentioned, this glide can be as little as 2–4 mm for the crease to indent inward under the overhanging lid fold,

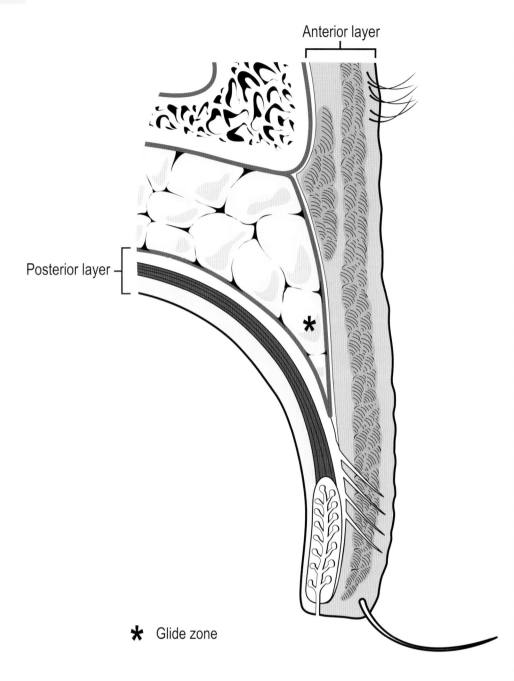

Anterior layer

Posterior layer

* Glide zone

Fig. 16-5 Concept of glide zone. The glide zone consists of the space occupied by the preaponeurotic fat pads, as well as all potential space between the anterior orbicularis oculi muscle–orbital septum layers and the posterior layers of the levator–levator aponeurosis–Müller's muscle–tarsal plate. The middle zone (glide zone) where the preaponeurotic fat pads are located acts like a frictionless lubricating layer which allows the posterior layer to glide upwards. When the patient looks from down to straight ahead with the eyelid open, the levator (agonist) contracts and the sphincter-like pretarsal, preseptal, and periorbital layers of the orbicularis relax. The orbicularis muscle of the upper lid is anchored at the medial and lateral canthal commissures, fusing there as a component of the medial and lateral canthal ligaments. The anterior layer therefore act like a passive layer, affected by gravity as the posterior layer of the active levator and Müller's muscle contracts to open the eyelid from a closed position. The up-vectoring of the semirigid tarsal plate therefore depends on the middle layer to allow it to hinge upwards against the passively resisting anterior layer to form an upper lid crease. The anterior layer glides passively over the posterior layer (upper part of the tarsal plate) for several millimeters in the process of forming the upper lid crease; the portion of skin overhanging the tarsal plate is the eyelid fold.

which consists of skin, orbicularis, and orbital septum arising from the arcus marginalis of the superior orbital rim. The anterior layer therefore hangs from the superior orbital rim and the area superficial to it, whereas the posterior layer originates from the orbital apex and contracts posterosuperiorly as it lies on the surface of the eye.

The typical findings immediately following a suboptimal aesthetic Asian lid crease procedure (using the external incision approach), as well as following traditional upper blepharoplasty in a non-Asian, may include an unusual amount of swelling (tissue edema, hemorrhage from orbicularis or any of the vascular arcades[11-14]), excessive removal of fat from the

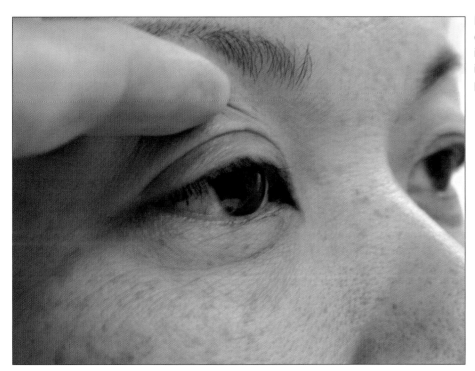

Fig. 16-6 Glide sign. The superficial dermis can glide over the deeper layers in a normal eyelid. An abnormal finding indicates adherence of the anterior and posterior layers.

preaponeurotic space (the third layer), and inadequate construction of the crease based on physiologic principles. As the swelling recedes, any of the following may appear: a lower than normal position of the upper lid margin (ptosis), a hollow sulcus, an absent or insufficient crease formation, and multiple creases (with or without a primary crease). These are all signs relating to inadequate management or excessive anatomic manipulation of tissues within the glide zone. By this I mean the obliteration of this glide space by aggressive fat excision, from cicatrization following excessive hemorrhage or handling within the preaponeurotic space, or adhesions involving the orbicularis, orbital septum, and levator aponeurosis. As healing progresses, the upper eyelid continues to manifest some degree of ptosis or resistance to upgaze, with poor crease invagination. The patient may complain of effort in keeping the lids open, difficulty gazing upward, and having a portion of the superior visual field obstructed. (With time, an initially restrictive-type ptosis may develop into an acquired ptosis with true weakening of the levator muscle.) The pretarsal as well as the preseptal eyelid skin may appear as a single zone of relatively flattened and convex plaque of thickened skin overlying the globe. This is indicated by one or all of the following:

- With the patient looking downward at the floor (not closing the eyelid fissure, as this encourages active contraction of the sphincter-like orbicularis muscle), the examiner applies his index finger gently and superficially over the midportion of the preseptal skin superior to the upper tarsus in order to push or glide the anterior skin–muscle layer superiorly (Fig. 16-6). If the layer fails to move upward for even 2 mm without the upper lid margin also moving upward, this is indicative of an abnormal 'glide sign'.

- With the patient looking downward, the examiner uses his thumb and index finger to try to pinch the preseptal zone's skin layer (above the tarsus) from the lid tissue underneath it (Fig. 16-7). An abnormal traction of the anterior layer, indicated by the posterior layer and upper eyelid margin also coming off the surface of the globe, is suggestive of an abnormal obliteration of the glide zone or preaponeurotic space, constituting an abnormal 'pinch sign'.

- With the patient looking down, the ipsilateral eyebrow splinted by the examiner's other hand to prevent brow action on upgaze, and the examiner pinching the preseptal skin, the patient is then

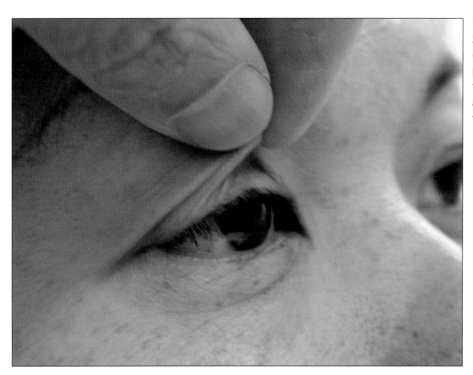

Fig. 16-7 Pinch sign. When the glide zone is intact, the preseptal skin–muscle (anterior) layer can be lifted over the posterior layers of the eyelid without the tarsus coming off of the globe. An abnormal finding indicates adherence of the anterior and posterior layers.

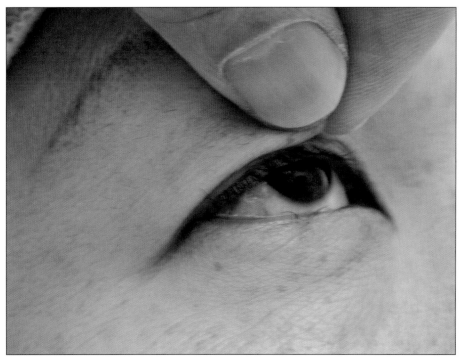

Fig. 16-8 Upgaze skin traction sign. The patient is asked to look up while the skin is secured by the examiner's fingers. Abnormal traction suggests adherence and obliteration of the preaponeurotic space or glide zone.

asked to look upward. As the patient looks up, the superior rectus and levator both contract. A normal finding would be the upper eyelid margin moving up independently without the pinched skin moving upward (Fig. 16-8). If the examiner's fingers feel an upward tug from the patient's pinched preseptal skin being pulled up also, it indicates that the posterior and anterior layers are fused together and is an abnormal 'upgaze skin traction sign'.

The above findings apply more to adults who have had surgery and not undergone significant involutional changes, and would not be accurate in those unlikely revisional cases where there is still excess residual skin in the preseptal area, or where there is age-related dehiscence between the preseptal skin and the underlying preseptal orbicularis oculi muscle, such that a false negative may occur (in a situation where, although the glide zone has been obliterated, it is still possible to glide, pinch the skin relative to the adherent orbicularis, and have no skin traction on upgaze). It is also possible that a patient with fused anterior and posterior layers may have a false-negative finding in any one or two of the above tests, but it is unlikely that all three would be 'normal' on evaluation. This combination of glide sign, pinch sign, and upgaze skin traction has been helpful for me and is an additional tool in the clinical assessment of patients with revision problems.

In revision attempts following suboptimal results, it is therefore crucial to be able to identify and reach this third space and recreate a glide zone if possible. At the same time, any scar tissue within this potential space can be approached and cleared, including the removal of any buried sutures. To correct for a hollowed supratarsal sulcus, it is logical to identify and re-establish this potential glide space and to supplement the deficient volume with a free fat graft.

In my previous paper on trapezoidal debulking of the preaponeurotic platform[7] it can be seen that the removal of skin and some orbicularis in a beveled fashion does not involve aggressive excision of the lower span of the orbital septum for more than several millimeters from the upper incisional skin border; the septum is merely opened to allow access. Upon wound closure, the edge of the orbital septum is still allowed to lie back on the anterior surface of the distal portion of the levator aponeurosis, at or slightly above the superior tarsal border, thereby preserving as well as forming the anterior boundary of this glide zone.

Other factors that will facilitate the construction of a crease include the excision of previous scar (provided there is sufficient skin in reserve), correction of ptosis, and correction of any factors impeding this glide (shift) of the posterior layer. Among the latter are maneuvers that clear any adhesion between the anterior and posterior layers. The skin–orbicularis layer may have been inadvertently laid on to the levator during

closure of the previous wounds, without proper positioning of the eyebrows and forehead owing to lack of proper loosening of the surgical drape on the forehead. The re-establishment of the glide zone, as well as downward and appropriate positioning of the anterior layer and the eyebrow–forehead complex, allows the now 'released' tarsal plate to be properly pulled by the freed posterior layer of the levator muscle, whose contraction then yields a crease superficial to the tarsal–aponeurotic junction along the superior tarsal border. This can be apparent as the patient lies on the operating table even without any sutures closing the skin edges together (Fig. 16-9).

In terms of what is seen preoperatively in any Asian patient undergoing a primary crease enhancement procedure, a typical creaseless Asian eyelid may present with one or more of the following: fullness in the pretarsal zone, an absence of skin invagination along the superior tarsal border (lack of an acute angle at the tarsoaponeurotic junction), fullness over the preaponeurotic/preseptal area, primary or secondary mild ptosis, as well as levator function that is on the low side of normal. The various methods of crease construction include the tightening of the tarsoaponeurotic junctional zone by suture ligation,[3] buried sutures, thermal cautery, external bead compression (the recently modified method of Shirakabe[6]), the partial incision methods with varying amount of soft tissue excision (including skin, orbicularis, and preaponeurotic fat) coupled with crease fixation using skin–aponeurosis attachment, buried orbicularis–levator aponeurosis fixation, or skin–tarsus fixation all work to some degree in facilitating the upward vectoring of the tarsus against the anterior eyelid layer to form the crease, provided the glide zone is preserved or has not been greatly disturbed during the incisional approach. Complications that are very challenging to correct often follow obliteration of the glide zone. During the relatively non-invasive techniques of transconjunctival or transcutaneous suturing, unexpected and sudden bleeding has been reported and may occur as a result of injury to the vertically oriented anastomotic vessels of the marginal and peripheral arcades of the upper lid,[11] as well as the deep orbital arcade,[12,13] and can also involve the recently described lateral septoaponeurotic artery found in a certain proportion of the population.[14] The bleeding may occur in the postaponeurotic plane if the vessels retract after the plane is transected

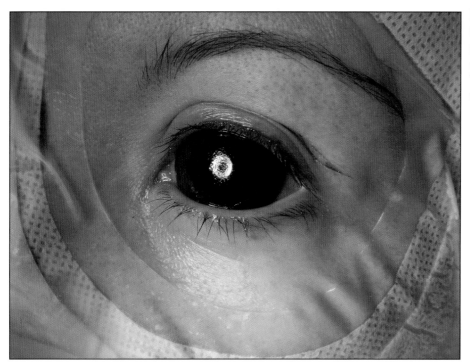

Fig. 16-9 Intraoperative appearance of the intraoperative crease form in a revision patient prior to the application of crease-fixation sutures and closure. The globe is protected by a black corneal protector.

in front of the tarsus or aponeurosis, or within the preaponeurotic space (the glide zone) itself. Residual adhesion may follow resolution of blood clots and lead to irregularity in the crease thus created, or to partial, segmental, or complete disappearance of the crease.

Summary

In conclusion, the eyelid crease is an anatomic invagination of the external skin along the superior tarsal border. It arises from a complex interaction of vector forces which in turn depend on the following: a healthy and unrestricted levator muscle; a firm upper tarsus and pretarsal platform; an adequate attachment of distal aponeurotic fibers towards the pretarsal orbicularis fibers, as well as the subcutaneous area beneath the crease; the presence of a third layer called the glide layer (which normally has preaponeurotic fat within it); the presence of non-rigid tissues in the preseptal region (supratarsal region) which rolls over passively as an eyelid fold over the invaginating crease; the absence of excess redundant tissues in the preseptal zone; the absence of skin shortage in this same preseptal area of the fold; the absence of rigid skin or scarring that may bond the anterior and posterior layers of the upper lid together; and a properly positioned eye-

brow. The theoretical basis for preservation of this third layer – the preaponeurotic glide zone and the role it plays in primary as well as revisional blepharoplasty – has been detailed in this chapter and should provide greater understanding in the management of all upper blepharoplasty and complex revisional issues.

References

1. Cheng J, Xu Feng-Zhi. Anatomic microstructure of the upper eyelid in the Oriental double eyelid. Plast Reconstruct Surg 2001;107:1665–1668.
2. Hwang K, Kim DJ, Chung RS, Lee SI, Hiraga Y. An anatomical study of the junction of the orbital septum and the levator aponeurosis in Orientals. Br J Plast Surg 1998;51:594–598.
3. Mutou Y, Mutou H. Intradermal double eyelid operation and its follow-up results. Br J Plast Surg 1972;25: 285–291.
4. Tsurukiri K. Double eyelid plasty: reliability and unfavorable results to the patients [Abstract]. J Jpn Aesth Plast Surg 1999;20:38.
5. Homma K, Mutou Y, Mutou H, Ezoe K, Fujita T. Intradermal stitch for Orientals: does it disappear? Aesth Plast Surg 2000;24:289–291.

6. Shirakabe Y. Mikamo's double-eyelid operation: The advent of Japanese aesthetic surgery (Discussion by Yukio Shirakabe MD). Plast Reconstruct Surg 1997;99: 668–669.

7. Chen WPD. Concept of triangular, rectangular and trapezoidal debulking of eyelid tissues: application in Asian blepharoplasty. Plast Reconstruct Surg 1996;97:212–218.

8. Khoo BC. Further experience with cosmetic surgery of the upper eyelid. Proceedings of the Third International Congress of Plastic Surgery. Excerpta Medica International Congress Series No.66:518–524,1963.

9. Khoo BC. Secondary blepharoplasty in Orientals. In: Khoo B-C. Problems in plastic reconstructive surgery. Vol.1. Philadelphia: JB Lippincott, 1991: 520–535.

10. Flowers RS. Upper blepharoplasty by eyelid invagination – anchor blepharoplasty. Clin Plast Surg 1993;20:193–207.

11. Kawai K, Imanishi N, Nakajima H et al. Arterial anatomic features of the upper palpebra. Plast Reconstruct Surg 2004;13:479–484.

12. Khoo BC. Perioperative bleeding in the pretarsal (post-aponeurotic) space in oriental blepharoplasty. Br J Plast Surg 2001;54:370.

13. Kim BG, Youn DY, Yoon ES et al. Unexpected bleeding caused by arterial variation inferolateral to levator palpebrae. Aesth Plast Surg 2003;27:123–125.

14. Hwang K, Kim BG, Kim YJ, Chung IH. Lateral septoaponeurotic artery: source of bleeding in blepharoplasty performed in Asians. Ann Plast Surg 2003;50:16–159.

Advanced Concepts: The Beveled Approach and Mid-Lemellar Clearance in Revisional Asian Blepharoplasty

Chapter 17

William P.D. Chen

The author has often advocated the trapezoidal debulking of the preaponeurotic platform using a beveled approach (along the upper incision line) in Asian blepharoplasty as a logical and efficient way of performing primary cases.[1-6] This approach offers the following advantages:

1. An easier and safer approach to the preaponeurotic space through the orbital septum when the plane of dissection is beveled.
2. A controlled, uniform debulking of junctional tissues overlying the preseptal (supratarsal) and pretarsal areas.
3. Optimal adhesions between levator aponeurosis and the subcutaneous tissues along the lower incision line, or to intermuscular septa within pretarsal orbicularis muscle fibers (pretarsal platform).
4. Crease formation can be based on the individual's tarsus height.
5. Virtual elimination of any potential for an uneven plane of surgical dissection, thereby lessening the complication rate, which include problems with asymmetry, height, shape, continuity, permanency, segmentation of the crease, fading and late disappearance of the crease, multiple creases, and persistent edema.

The clinical findings seen in patients seeking revisional surgery are myriad. The eyelid may show spreading of the incision scar, high placement of the crease, induced lagophthalmos on downgaze, and acquired secondary ptosis on straight gaze as well as upgaze. Intraoperatively, one sees thickened middle lamellar scar involving the orbicularis oculi as well as the orbital septum, or the presence of dense scar tissue plaques that may bind the anterior orbicularis oculi as well as the posterior levator aponeurosis (Fig. 17-1). Instead of having a physiologically preserved 'glide zone' where significant preaponeurotic fat pads are still present in the lowest aspect of the glide space, there is now a con-

densed apron (plaque) of tissue that is preventing the posterior layer from up-vectoring properly against a passive and flexible skin–orbicularis layer. Despite all efforts, there is no observable crease formation. Patients often complain of lid fatigue, a feeling of tightness, and may show brow and forehead overaction.

In dealing with revision cases, whether simple or complicated, one of the greatest dilemmas is where to make the incision so that it does not compound the already scarred field of operation, both from an anterior skin viewpoint (and therefore an aesthetic concern) and as regards middle lamellar scarring and contracture (with further functional compromise). To succeed with improved aesthetic results as well as without further functional setbacks is a major triumph for any surgeon familiar with and undertaking this type of revision surgery. Not only is the operation difficult, but often the patient is anxious for a rapid and successful outcome, something that is never easily realized when dealing with scarring and suboptimal outcomes. I am often struck by how devastated these patients are and how grateful when the improvement proves significant. It is important for both patient and surgeon to be realistic in their expectations, as well as their projection of the time course of healing following revisional surgery.

Having said that, the following are the minimal requirements in revisional surgery that I have striven for in my practice:

1. That we do not cause further skin shortage.
2. That we do not cause increased midlamellar contraction, with lid retraction and poor eyelid closure.
3. That neither of the two factors above leads to consecutive symptoms of exposure and dryness of the ocular surface.
4. That the patient understands from the first that the physician will not be able to achieve a level of aesthetic improvement rivaling that of the primary cases in his practice, where conditions are ideal,

255

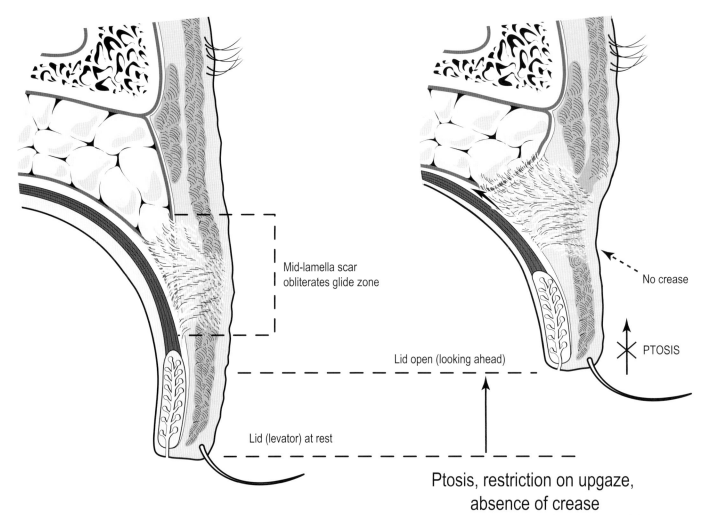

Mid-lamella scar
obliterates glide zone

No crease

PTOSIS

Lid open (looking ahead)

Lid (levator) at rest

Ptosis, restriction on upgaze,
absence of crease

Fig. 17-1 Scarring seen in suboptimal cases of aesthetic surgery of the Asian upper eyelid may include spreading of the incisional skin, high placement of the crease, induced lagophthalmos on downgaze, and acquired secondary ptosis on straight gaze as well as upgaze. Intraoperatively, one sees middle lamellar scar involving the orbicularis oculi as well as the orbital septum, or the presence of dense scar tissue plaques that may bind the anterior orbicularis oculi as well as the posterior levator aponeurosis. Instead of having a physiologically preserved 'glide zone' where preaponeurotic fat pads are still present in the lowest aspect of the glide space, there is now a condensed apron-like plaque of tissue that is preventing the posterior layer from up-vectoring properly against a passive and flexible skin–orbicularis layer. Despite all efforts, there is no observable crease formation. Patients often complain of fatigue, a feeling of tightness, and may show brow and forehead overaction.

the amount of skin is adequate, and patient expectations closer to being normal and fair.

5. That the patient be informed that for each revision operation one can try to correct only one item from a list of goals. By this I mean that it is impossible, for example, to correct an abnormally high crease, lid margin contour deformity, pre-existing ptosis, and a shortage of skin all at the same time.

All these factors funnel into the same conclusion: if there is insufficient skin in reserve, it is unlikely that

there is any chance of revisional improvement unless one wishes to supplement the skin with a free full-thickness skin graft. This latter will require precise techniques, experience, and special splinting over the graft in order to place it in an aesthetically acceptable fashion. There are, however, many young adults or middle-aged patients who need revisional surgery, whose problems are severe and who are unlikely to have any skin reserves in the future because of natural aging. Patients with just enough eyelid closure to avoid corneal exposure can develop such symptoms if the usual method of excision of the scar and lysis of adhe-

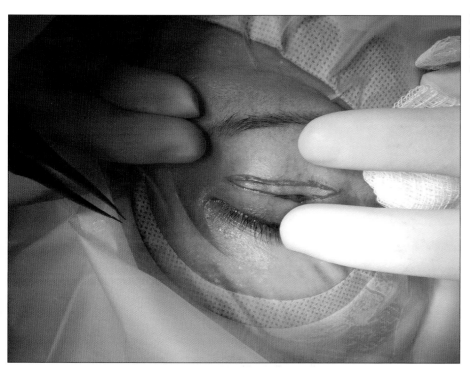

Fig. 17-2 A full-thickness skin incision has been made along the upper and lower lines of the crease marking (left upper lid).

sion of the middle lamella is followed. The amount of skin removed can be as little as 2 mm, and poor eyelid closure can be the result.

An ideal solution to this dilemma is to approach the scarred anterior and middle lamellar complex through a superiorly beveled approach. To do this, the following conditions must be met.

The crease height is evaluated, and if it is high then the degree of planned lowering (in millimeters) will determine the minimum amount of skin redundancy above the existing crease (over the preseptal region) that needs to be in reserve. For example, if the suboptimal crease is currently at 10.5 mm and you plan to lower it to 7.5 mm, then the patient will need to have 3 mm of skin in reserve above the crease before this is feasible. If there is only 2 mm, then this needs to be discussed with the patient, as the crease can only be revised down to 8.5 mm in the current situation, or the patient can opt to wait for some skin to become available as a result of natural aging (and they may proceed to revision at that time). If this cannot be achieved and the patient is desperate, for either functional or psychological reasons, then one must discuss the option of a free skin graft.

For the majority who may be candidates for revision without the need for skin grafting, my surgical approach proceeds initially along the same path as in primary cases, the major exception being that the upper and lower incision lines are marked directly next to each other on either side of the existing scar. Patients in this category are more likely to have had their lid crease incision made in the 8–9 mm range, as measured from the central lid margin. The separation of the upper and lower incision lines should be no more than 1 mm, and very rarely 2 mm. A no.15 Bard–Parker blade is used to make a full-thickness incision along the marked upper and lower lines (Fig. 17-2). Now, instead of using cutting cautery to go through the orbicularis to reach the orbital septum, one uses a sharp-tipped Westcott spring scissors to incise across the upper line of incision in a superiorly beveled fashion (Fig. 17-3). At this stage, it is cutting through skin-orbicularis adhesions. Small scissoring motions are then used as the scissor blades transect the middle lamellar scar, opening through the whitish, scarred fascial layers between the orbicularis and the underlying levator aponeurosis (Fig. 17-4). This is carried out through the width of the incision along the previous scar. The beveled approach is quite similar, but steeper than in primary cases (Fig. 17-5). In this scarred middle zone there will be much less preaponeurotic fat, as it will have been previously excised; some residual fat globules, combined with scattered smaller amorphous globules or aprons of scattered fat droplets, may be seen

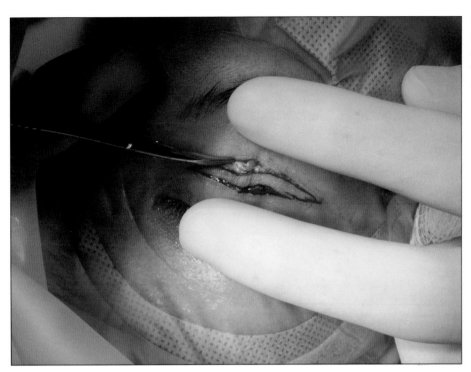

Fig. 17-3 Westcott spring scissors are used to lyze along the upper incisional edge in a beveled fashion. It is cutting through skin-orbicularis adhesions (left upper lid).

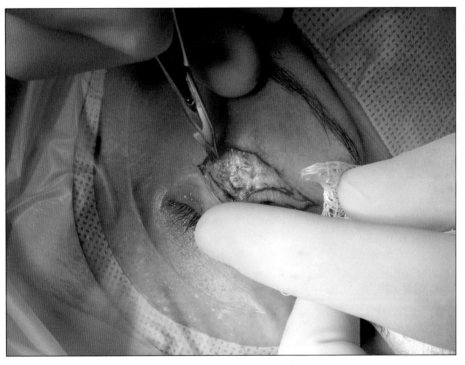

Fig. 17-4 Small scissoring motions are applied as the scissor blades transect the middle lamellar scar, going through whitish, scarred fascial layers between the orbicularis and the underlying levator aponeurosis (left upper lid).

(Fig. 17-6). The scarred tissues in the anterior layer as well as in the mid-lamellar zone – encompassed by the tissues between the dotted superiorly beveled vector in the figure and the lower skin incision (along the superior tarsal border) – may be excised after the forehead/eyebrow/preseptal skin layers are carefully reset (by releasing any restrictive surgical adhesive or drapes on the patient's forehead), for as long as the remaining skin still allows passive eyelid closure. All fat is preserved. The levator and levator aponeurosis can be identified when the scar is released, and it is important to check for restriction objectively (by gently pulling the tarsal plate down) as well as subjectively by asking the patient to perform upgaze and

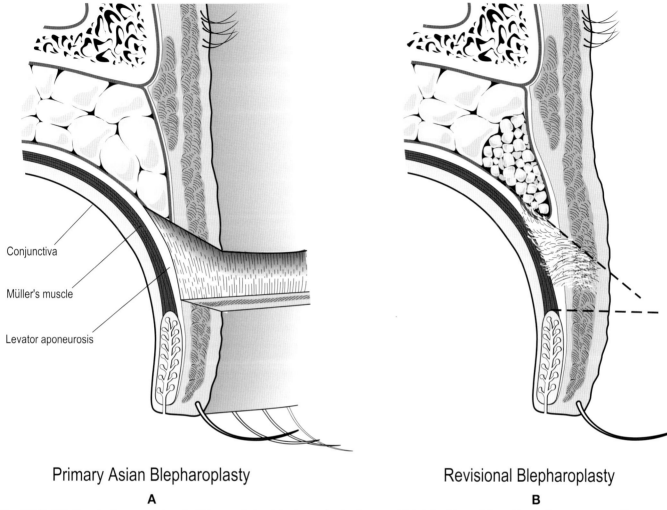

Conjunctiva

Müller's muscle

Levator aponeurosis

Primary Asian Blepharoplasty

A

Revisional Blepharoplasty

B

Fig. 17-5 (A) Beveled approaches in Primary Asian blepharoplasty: trapezoidal debulking of the skin and preaponeurotic platform. **(B)** Superiorly beveled approach in revisional Asian blepharoplasty. Note the gentler beveled approach used in primary case versus the much steeper (oblique) approach taken in revisional attempts. This is necessary in the latter situation to preserve skin and to allow identification of the former preaponeurotic zone. In this scarred middle zone one frequently finds some residual larger fat pads combined with scattered smaller amorphous fat globules or aprons of scattered fat droplets. The scarred tissues in the anterior layer as well as the mid-lamellar zone, encompassed by the tissues between the dotted superiorly beveled vector in the drawing and the lower skin incision (along the superior tarsal border), may be excised after the forehead/eyebrow/preseptal skin layers are carefully reset, for as long as the remaining skin allows passive eyelid closure. All fat is preserved.

downgaze. The benefits and advantages of this approach are as follows:

1. By approaching the preaponeurotic space very close to and barely superior to the suboptimal scarred crease line, one can avoid taking out a precious 0.5 or 1 mm of good skin.
2. By making the upper line of incision close to the scarred crease line, one avoids creating an extra incisional scar.

3. This beveled approach to the previously explored preaponeurotic space allows the space to be entered safely again, without injury to underlying levator muscle and Müller's muscle, as well as avoiding any anastomotic vascular arcades in Müller's muscle and the superior tarsal arteriolar arcade.
4. In some cases, this beveled maneuver towards the preaponeurotic space frees up the vertical excursion of the upper eyelid significantly,

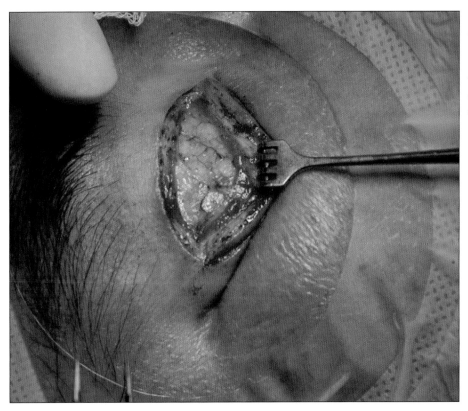

Fig. 17-6 After the preaponeurotic space is reached, within this scarred middle zone one frequently finds some residual larger fat globules combined with scattered smaller amorphous fat globules or aprons of scattered fat droplets (right upper lid).

releasing any restriction that may have contributed to lagophthalmos and acquired ptosis. This maneuver in itself may correct the mild ptosis, such that resetting of the previously high crease is then feasible.

5. Approaching the preaponeurotic space in any revisional upper blepharoplasty allows one to identify residual preaponeurotic fat that may have spread out and become plastered down on the levator muscle. This residual fat can be peeled off and repositioned at a higher level within the sulcus to help reverse some of the hollow sulcus often seen in patients needing revisional blepharoplasty.

6. Mid-lamellar scarring that has previously bonded the anterior and posterior layers can be safely removed or reduced, allowing partial restoration of the glide zone.

Following revisional Asian blepharoplasty using a superiorly beveled approach, the glide space has been partially restored and the scar carefully removed (Fig. 17-7). The preaponeurotic platform is cleared of any interfering tissues. Although the surgeon is often forced to make a skin incision that is still further from the lid margin than one would for a primary Asian blepharoplasty, upon closure the incision wound (white dot) is free to indent inwards when the levator contracts, forming a better crease. The residual fat pads in the middle (glide) zone are preserved and allowed to fill in this space where appropriate. (In severe cases a fat graft may be considered in this space.) Skin denoted by the red and blue dots above the incision is now free to hang down and around to form the contrasting eyelid fold.

Dynamics of The Upper Eyelid Crease

In a traditional approach to primary upper blepharoplasty the upper and lower lines of incision are normally made with the surgical blade perpendicular (90°) to the skin. The skin, muscle, and preaponeurotic fat are reduced by excision in an appropriate fashion. Upon closure of the wound and reformation of the crease (incision line closure), the preaponeurotic space is allowed to be set inferiorly and now reaches an area over the superior tarsal border. Three scenarios follow.

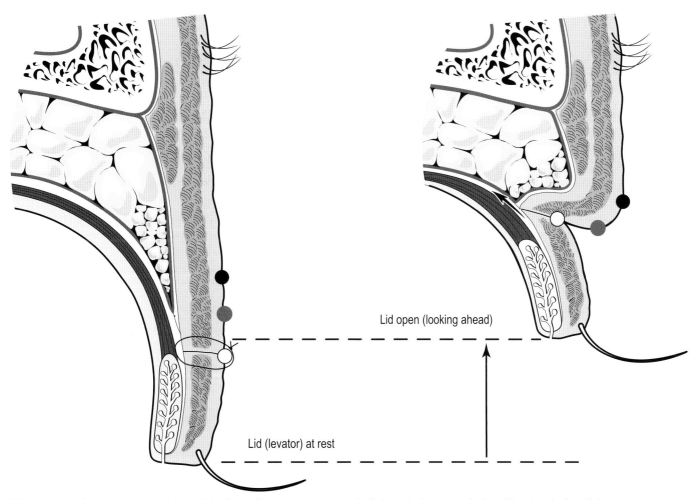

Fig. 17-7 Following revisional Asian blepharoplasty using a superiorly beveled approach (see Fig. 17-5), the glide space has been partially restored and the scar removed. The preaponeurotic platform is cleared of any interfering tissues. Although the surgeon is often forced to make a skin incision that is still further from the lid margin than one would for a primary Asian blepharoplasty, upon closure the incision wound (white dot) is free to indent inwards when the levator contracts, forming a better crease. The residual fat pads in the middle (glide) zone are preserved and allowed to fill in this glide space where appropriate. Skin denoted by the black and gray dots above the incision is now free to hang down and around to form the contrasting eyelid fold.

1. If the exposed preaponeurotic fat was completely excised, what remains of the septum and overlying preseptal orbicularis is now lying over and directly in contact with the levator aponeurosis, with no fat buffering. There is a good chance that the preaponeurotic space (glide zone) will be obliterated. The result is a deep-set supratarsal sulcus as well as poor crease formation.

2. If there were only partial or conservative removal of fat, there is the possibility that some fat will still be interposed between the preseptal orbicularis muscle (anterior layer) and the aponeurosis (posterior layer).

3. In my beveled approach towards the upper incision line, upon surgical closure of the incision the upper skin edge alone is attached to aponeurosis along the superior tarsal border as well as the lower skin edge; there is also preservation of the preaponeurotic space and fat down to the superior tarsal border, coupled with some fat buffering in the glide zone. More orbicularis fibers are removed along the upper incisional edge, as the orbicularis was transected in an upwardly beveled fashion. This allows the immediate vicinity of the upper incisional skin edge to be in contact with the preaponeurotic space thus created.

In the last two situations, where fat was only partially excised (or repositioned superiorly), whether via a traditional rectangular debulking of the preaponeurotic platform or via a trapezoidal debulking of the soft tissues, the preaponeurotic space over the preseptal mid-region of the upper lid has been preserved. There is fat buffering (preservation of the preaponeurotic space or glide zone) as well as a soft tissue mass (consisting of the preseptal skin, orbicularis, orbital septum, and preaponeurotic fat) bellowing on top of a dynamically elevating tarsal plate. The redundant soft tissue platform (previously referred to as preaponeurotic platform) has been reduced by an appropriate amount. The crease formed is dynamic and natural from an aesthetic viewpoint.

The restoration and preservation of the preaponeurotic space is an essential element in the surgical creation of a crease for an Asian with a creaseless eyelid, for it is the up-vectoring of the tarsal plate, coupled with the attendant presence of fat in the preserved preaponeurotic space, that helps create the appearance of a well formed crease under a preseptal eyelid fold contour of the mid-section of the upper eyelid.

It would be undesirable to completely excise fat, thereby obliterating the preaponeurotic space, flatten the preseptal mid-section, and create a supratarsal sulcus on an Asian upper lid.

The following reasoning is applied to revisional blepharoplasty. By utilizing the *superiorly beveled* approach along the upper line of incision, I aim to preserve the integrity of the preaponeurotic space. If the patient has previously undergone a traditional *rectangular debulking* with partial excision of fat, this approach will allow one to locate the preaponeurotic space without much difficulty. If the previous surgeon carried out the *trapezoidal debulking* method,[1] it is relatively easy to find the preaponeurotic space, as I do when performing touch-up enhancement of the crease. If the patient has undergone rectangular debulking with *total fat removal*, the beveled approach still gives a greater chance of reaching a familiar surgical landscape, that is, the preaponeurotic space. (The fourth scenario of trapezoidal debulking with complete fat removal has not so far been encountered by this author, as most surgeons nowadays know not to remove too much fat in Asian eyelids; however, not so many are familiar with trapezoidal debulking using a beveled approach as applied to Asians.)

Often a patient will present with a history of upper lid aesthetic surgery and exhibit a flattened or absent crease with a mild hollowing of the sulcus. The patient may have poor crease formation for a number of reasons, including poor surgical adhesion between the skin edges and the aponeurosis, or the presence of an amorphous sheet of fat that appears plastered down over the entire aponeurosis within the preaponeurotic space between skin and levator.

The beveled approach as applied in revisional Asian blepharoplasty allows the surgeon to reach the preaponeurotic space safely, to reposition any remaining preaponeurotic fat superiorly to fill in the hollow, and to approach the preaponeurotic space without having to sacrifice precious millimeters of skin along the upper skin incision line through excision. In other words, you are making sure that your incision will not add to the problem, while allowing yourself access to the eyelid's preaponeurotic space to excise middle lamellar scar, re-establish a glide interface, and to recreate a relatively physiologic and dynamic crease (Fig. 17-8A and B).

Scarring seen in suboptimal cases of aesthetic surgery of the Asian upper eyelid may include spreading of the incisional skin, high placement of the lid crease, induced lagophthalmos on downgaze, and acquired secondary ptosis on straight gaze as well as upgaze. Intraoperatively, one sees middle lamellar scar involving the orbicularis oculi as well as the orbital septum, or the presence of dense scar tissue plaques that may bind the anterior orbicularis oculi as well as the posterior levator aponeurosis. Instead of having a physiologically preserved 'glide zone' where preaponeurotic fat pads are still present in the lowest aspect of the glide space, there is now a condensed apron (plaque) of tissue preventing the posterior layer from upvectoring properly against a passive and flexible skin–orbicularis layer.

Within the author's practice, a series[7] of 26 patients and 48 eyelids underwent revisional blepharoplasty over the last four years for the specific purpose of revising a post-surgical high crease to a lower position. Excluded from this series were all primary Asian Blepharoplasty including any patients with pre-existent high crease, touch-up surgery for the purpose of enhancing (deepening) an existing or surgically-created crease, correction of incomplete crease or crease shape alone, and simultaneous correction of acquired or involutional ptosis in conjunction with primary Asian blepharoplasty.

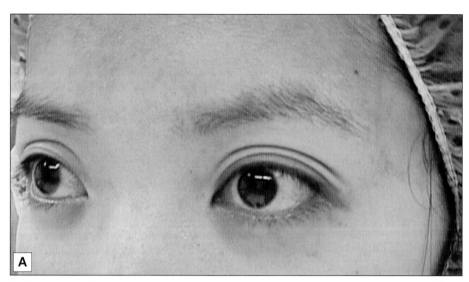

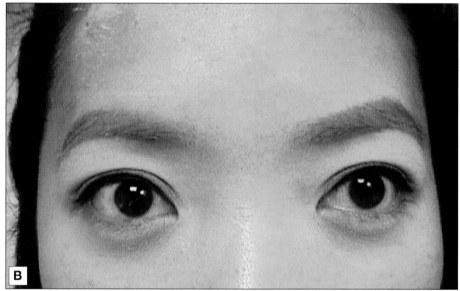

Fig. 17-8 (A) Preoperative appearance prior to revision. **(B)** Postoperative appearance after revision.

There were 5 males and 21 females, and with the exception of four patients who requested unilateral crease revisions, all others were bilateral.

The data was arranged in two separate sets of columns. OD for the right upper lid, OS for the left upper lid. The third column of each of these two clusters of data reflects the difference between the preoperative and postoperative measurements. There were 24 eyelids in each category, for a total of 48 eyelids. The data were pooled together to arrive at the overall statistical mean. The pre-revisional crease height was measured in the office using a millimeter scale and ranges between 8–14 mm, with the overall mean being 9.9 mm. The crease height designed during revision (in 0.5 mm increments) varied between 6.0–8.5 mm based on the circumstances, with the mean being 7.15 mm;

and 7 mm was the most often applied measurement during surgery under local anesthetic. The effective lowering of the crease height ranges from one to six millimeters when reassessed during their two months post-revisional visits. The mean lowering of crease height is 2.75 mm in this series based on two months followup. The typical course is such that the crease height will continue to settle down with egress of swelling and wound healing, such that the effective lowering of the crease will likely increase had it been possible for all these patients to return for a lengthtier followup period.

(The above data is abridged from a paper submitted to and accepted for publication by the Journal of Plastic and Reconstructive Surgery, titled: 'The Bevelled Approach in Revisional Upper Blepharoplasty').

	Age & Gender	Preop OD	Postop OD	CHANGE	Preop OS	Postop OS	CHANGE
1	42F	12	7.5	4.5	11	7.5	3.5
2	38F	11	7.5	3.5	10	7.5	2.5
3	46F	11	7	4	10	7	3
4	60F	10	6	4	10	6	4
5	54F	9.5	7.5	2	9.5	7.5	2
6	32F	9	7	2	9	7	2
7	32F				8.5	6.5	2
8	22F	8.5	7	1.5	8.5	7	1.5
9	23M	8	7	1	8	7	1
10	63F	9	7	2	9	7	2
11	36F	12	8	4	14	8	6
12	58F	12	7	5	12	7	5
13	65F	11	7	4	11	7	4
14	29F	9	7	2	9	7	2
15	22F	9	8	1	9	8	1
16	55F	10	7.5	2.5	10	7.5	2.5
17	66F	9	6	3	8.5	6	2.5
18	30F	11	8.5	2.5	10	8	2
19	34F	9.5	8	1.5			
20	25F	8.5	7	1.5	8.5	7	1.5
21	39F	9	7	2	9	7	2
22	47F	11	8	3	11	8	3
23	28F				8	6.5	1.5
24	63F	10	7	3			
25	26F	9.5	6.5	3	9.5	6.5	3
26	28F	12	6	6	12	8	4
Subtotal =		240.5	172	68.5	235	171.5	63.5
Statis. Mean =		10.02	7.17	2.85	9.79	7.15	2.65
Total (OD + OS) =		475.5	343.5	132			
Overall Mean =		9.9	7.15	2.75			

Fig. 17-9 Revisional data in a series of 48 eyelids showing age, gender and degree of lowering of crease height in millimeters.

The use of a superiorly beveled approach in revisional Asian blepharoplasty can allow the glide zone to be partially restored and the middle lamellar scar removed. The preaponeurotic platform can be cleared of any interfering tissues. The combination of techniques described in this chapter often allows an abnormally high and static scar line to be repositioned into a lower and more dynamic crease, to the point of being acceptable for the patient. The need for skin grafting may often be avoided.

References

1. Chen WPD. Concept of triangular, rectangular and trapezoidal debulking of eyelid tissues: application in Asian blepharoplasty. Plast Reconstruct Surg 1996;971:212–218.

2. Chen WPD. Asian blepharoplasty: a surgical atlas. Oxford: Butterworth–Heinemann, 1995.

3. Chen WPD. Asian blepharoplasty – update on anatomy and technique. J Ophthalmol Plast Reconstruct Surg 1987;3:135–140.

4. Chen WPD. Aesthetic eyelid surgery in Asians: An east-west view. Hong Kong J Ophthalmol 2000;3:27–31.

5. Chen WPD. Oculoplastic surgery – the essentials. Stuttgart: Thieme, 2001.

6. Chen WPD, Khan J, McCord C. Color atlas of cosmetic oculofacial surgery. Oxford: Butterworth–Heinemann, 2004.

7. Chen WPD. The bevelled approach in revisional upper blepharoplasty. Plast Reconstruct Surg (publication pending).

Asian Eyelid Surgery: My Thoughts

Khoo Boo-Chai

Chapter 18

Khoo Boo-Chai of Singapore, a pioneer in this field since the 1960s, has kindly furnished all the information in this chapter, which has been abstracted by WPD Chen and reviewed by Dr. Boo-Chai. This is based on his 40 years of hands-on experience with aesthetic (cosmetic) surgery of the upper eyelid.

Boo-Chai[1] reported on his experience over 5 years with 625 cases of Asian lid crease procedures using the conjunctival stitch method. He recommended that this procedure is best used in patients with little upper lid fat and without a heavy fold that hangs down over the lid margin. Non-absorbable suture materials are used to connect the levator aponeurosis to the eyelid skin at a desired level 5–8 mm from the lid margin. If there is excessive supraorbital (preaponeurotic) fat, it is first removed through an additional central skin incision about one-quarter the width of the crease line designed.

The lid is everted and treated locally with 5% topical lidocaine solution; 0.5 mL of 1% lidocaine is given subconjunctivally. A needle bearing 4/0 nylon suture is passed through the conjunctiva in a horizontal fashion for 2–3 mm over the superior tarsal border. Each arm is then repassed through the conjunctiva towards the skin side overlying it. One arm of the externalized skin stitch is then passed subcutaneously towards the second arm, which is often itself passed through a small stab incision on the skin to facilitate the passage and subsequent burying of the knot. The two ends are tied, and the knot is tied down and buried under the skin surface. Usually three of these pairs of stitches are used.

Boo-Chai evaluated his patients 1 month postoperatively using the following parameters for a perfect result:

1. The creases on both sides must match in position, height, length, and contour.
2. The position and contour of the upper lid margin must match, without any notching or peaking.
3. The eyelashes must not be distorted or missing.
4. Blinking must be normal.

5. Both eyelids must close normally during sleep.
6. There must be minimal scarring and no ectropion.
7. The results must be permanent.

According to Boo-Chai, the advantages of this method include reversibility, minimal swelling, and the absence of an external linear scar.

Boo-Chai[2] also discussed the correction of the following three conditions: discrepancies in the height or shape of the crease, the absence of crease formation ('failed double-eyelid operation'), and a hollowed supratarsal recess due to excess removal of fat. In the introductory paragraphs he commented on the two main types of technique: the non-incisional suture techniques versus the incisional techniques with clearing of skin, fat, and use of skin–levator–skin fixation.

In the first category, when revising a previous non-incisional technique to eliminate discrepancies in crease height and shape, it is important to eliminate the crease by removing the loops of suture material that connected the levator to the skin. Boo-Chai prefers to apply the new crease-forming sutures usually three at the same setting after the previous loops have been removed.

For those with crease height and contour problems as a result of previous incisional techniques, he discussed two options:

1. If the patient wants an excessively low or shielded crease (caused by residual excess skin) to be corrected to a higher level to match the opposite side, Boo-Chai starts along the existing crease scar and designs an upper line of incision several millimeters above this. The excess skin is excised and the crease reconstructed.
2. In situations where there is no excess skin, he prefers to use a non-incisional buried suture loop technique to create the new higher crease without forming a second skin cut or scar.

He eliminates the previously created crease by going through the small stab incisions (used for the non-incisional method) and effectively undermining the adhesion between the aponeurosis and the dermis. The dissolution of this crease is verified intraoperatively by having the patient look upwards.

He also discussed lowering creases if both sides are higher than optimal, the emphasis being to include the existing scar line within the tissues to be excised.

In the second category, correction of poor crease formation, the revision involves excision of the previous fibrous tissue connection between levator and skin, as well as excision of the previous incisional scar. He then uses six or seven 4/0 sutures to connect skin to levator to skin.

The third category of revisional blepharoplasty involves the correction of a deepened sulcus caused by excess fat removal. Boo-Chai uses fat harvested from a lower blepharoplasty and the fat is then divided into numerous 3×4mm pellets. These are then placed behind the anterior layer of the orbital septum on top of the levator aponeurosis (with its closely attached posterior layer/reflection of orbital septum). He prefers to place more fat over the medial side of the upper lid. He notes that when observed 6 months later, these fat pellets seemed to have coalesced to form one piece.[3]

Boo-Chai[3] described the occasional presence of a marginal arterial arcade with perforating branches that pierce the levator aponeurosis near the insertion of the aponeurosis on the tarsus. These perforating vessels run perpendicularly in a vertical fashion, and lie within the suborbicularis areolar fatty tissues. They are not common and are difficult to detect unless specifically sought. When the lower skin flap is surgically manipulated or cleared, these perforators may be damaged and bleed, retracting within the aponeurosis to lie close to the marginal arterial arcade in the pretarsal (postaponeurotic) space, giving rise to a hematoma. Boo-Chai observed this in three cases, with an incidence of 1 in 500 cases. He went on to explain that the marginal arterial arcade normally lies on the tarsus 3mm from the lid margin. It receives a contribution medially from the superior medial palpebral branch of the ophthalmic artery and laterally from a branch of the lacrimal artery. In Asians, the marginal arterial arcade is covered by the levator aponeurosis, owing to its low insertion on the tarsus. This is in contrast to Caucasians, where the marginal arcade is not covered by the aponeurosis because its insertion is high up on the upper part of the tarsus. He stated that his pre-

ferred management of bleeding in such incidents was to apply ice compresses, and that the bleeding is self-limiting. He has subsequently called this form of bleeding the 'Boo-Chai sign'. It is unusual in the sense that the bleeding occurs suddenly posterior to the levator aponeurosis, and spreads widely within an area not usually touched during incisional methods of Asian eyelid surgery (Fig. 18-1 A,B).

Dr Boo-Chai's Personal Comments:

'In 2001, besides describing its clinical features for the first time in the *British Journal of Plastic Surgery*,[3] I also postulated its causation. I surmised that it was due to damage to an abnormally large branch of the marginal arterial arcade. That was only an educated guess, because the detailed anatomy of the vasculature of the upper eyelid was not then available in an anatomy text.

Two years after this publication, in 2003, a group of Korean plastic surgeons independently confirmed the clinical features of this bleeding complication in 25 of their cases.[4] They postulated that the bleeding occurred from damage to a blood vessel lying in the inferolateral part of the levator palpebrae. As to the exact vessel, they said that their research was ongoing and that they would publish a report as soon as they had arrived at a definitive conclusion.

Unbeknown to me and to them, however, a group of Japanese anatomists and plastic surgeons[5] performed a detailed anatomic study of the vasculature of the upper eyelid in seven Asian cadavers. They published their findings in 2004 in the *Journal of Plastic and Reconstructive Surgery*. This study confirmed my findings of the arrangement of the blood vessels and that the source of the mysterious bleeding was from an abnormally large branch of the marginal arterial arcade. Their study showed (a) that there are four arterial arcades in the upper lid, one lying about 3mm from the margin (marginal arcade), to which I had called attention; (b) the other, the peripheral arcade, is situated at the upper border of the tarsal plate (the other two are the superficial and deep orbital arcades, and they communicate with the marginal arterial arcade); (c) the arcades are interconnected by thin vertically oriented vessels. The small vertical branches running between the marginal and peripheral arcades, as well as that between the marginal arcade and the deep orbital arcade, lie in a plane posterior to the orbicularis oculi muscle. This also confirms my previous observations during surgery.

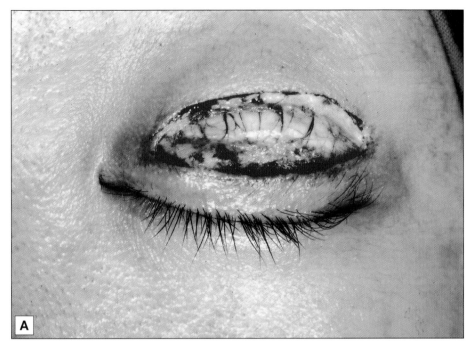

A

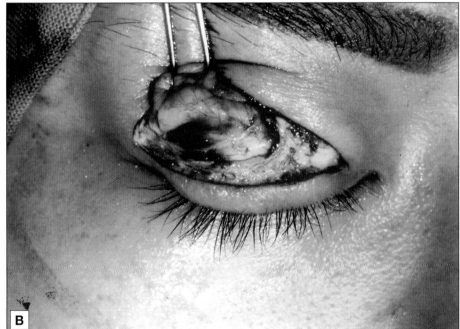

B

Fig. 18-1 (A) Left upper eyelid of a 25-year-old Chinese woman undergoing Asian blepharoplasty. A strip of skin and orbicularis oculi has been removed from the left upper lid, revealing giant branches of the marginal arcade running vertically upward. These branches emerge from underneath the anterior extent of the distal portion of the aponeurosis on the tarsal plate, and pierce the levator aponeurosis. They then course up vertically and lie in the retromuscular (suborbicularis) fat. Accidental damage to these branches when dissecting the skin flap will give rise to bleeding, with the formation of a hematoma behind and deep to the levator aponeurosis: the 'Boo-Chai sign'. **(B)** Right upper eyelid illustrating a self-limiting hematoma forming posterior to the levator aponeurosis.

I stated that very rarely a few (two or three) of these fine vertically running vessels become larger, penetrating the overlying levator aponeurosis and lying within the suborbicularis oculi fat. This was confirmed in the Japanese paper, which showed that the two arterial arcades are interconnected by vertically running vessels. When any of these abnormal branches of the marginal arcade are damaged during surgery, they can retract and end up lying posterior to the levator aponeurosis, resulting in a hematoma there.[3–5']

The Boo-Chai Method

The following is a step-by-step description of Boo-Chai's conjunctival suture method, as currently

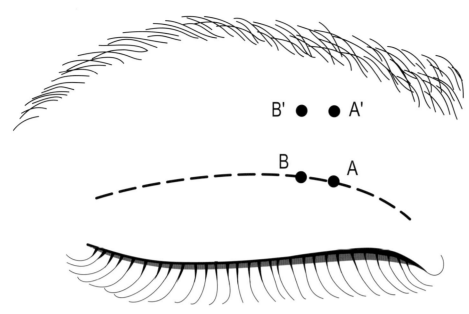

Fig. 18-2 Points A and B are on the lid skin side, 4–5 mm apart. A' and B' are on the conjunctival side 6 mm superior to points A and B, and are also 4–5 mm apart. The conjunctival surface is moist and difficult to mark with ink. The lid is everted gently with forceps or with the forefinger, and 0.5 mL of xylocaine are applied locally through the conjunctiva. This provides anesthesia as well as turgidity to the conjunctiva for easier passage of the needle (right upper lid).

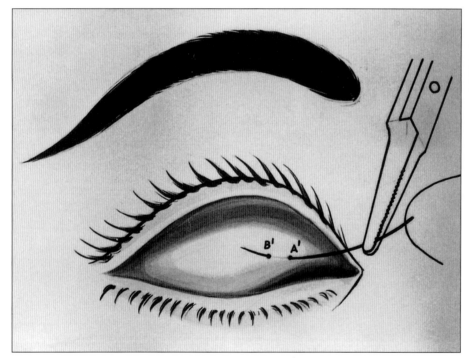

Fig. 18-3 Using a curved non-cutting needle (14–16 mm diameter) and either 4/0 or 5/0 nylon sutures the needle is passed from A' to B' subconjunctivally just beneath the surface and exiting through B' (right upper lid).

practiced by him (2006) in approximately 5–10% of his Asian patients seeking placement of an upper eyelid crease (Figs 18-2–18-7).

Principle

Using exogenous monofilament nylon slings to connect the levator palpebrae superioris to the eyelid skin at a desired level.

Medications and Instruments

Local anesthetic, 1–2% xylocaine with 1:100 000 dilution epinephrine; intravenous sedation as needed. Needle holder, three strands of 4/0 or 5/0 monofilament nylon, to be applied on a 14–16 mm curved, tapering non-cutting needle with an eyelet.

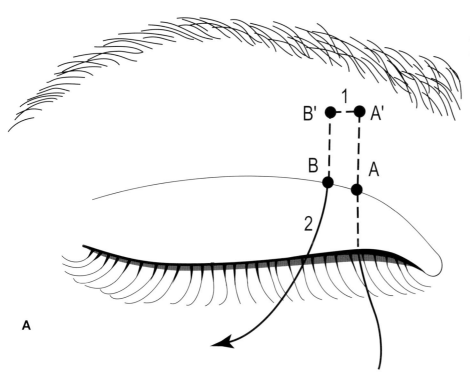

Fig. 18-4 (A, B) The needle coming out of B' is regripped and passed through B on the skin side in a trans-lid fashion (right upper lid).

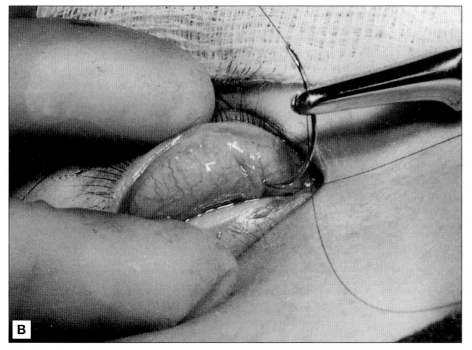

The desired level of the eyelid crease is marked with indelible ink on the skin side. It is important for the levels on both sides to be exactly the same, otherwise, at the end of the operation one may notice asymmetry, which is the most common cause of suboptimal results. The half-moon shaped crease is very popular. To achieve this using three slings, the middle sling should be about 2–3 mm higher than the other two.

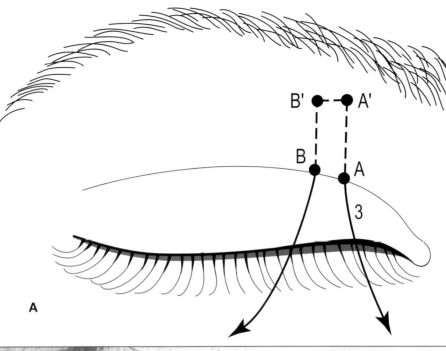

Fig. 18-5 (A, B) The needle itself is removed from the suture at B, and used to rethread the other end of the same suture coming from A'. It is similarly passed through the lid and exits through A on the skin side (right upper lid).

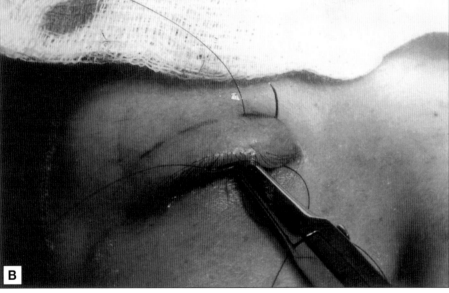

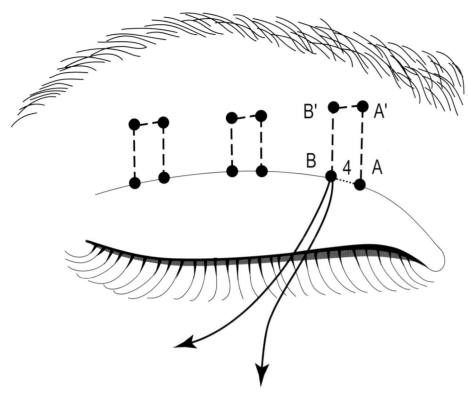

Fig. 18-6 Using the needle at A, the suture is passed subcutaneously towards B. This is repeated for the other two sets of nylon slings. With light pressure, check to verify that they are all in place. The tying is done only when all three sets of slings are in place, as it is difficult to evert the lids once the ends are tied. To facilitate the tied knot being buried under the skin surface at B, one may elect to make a small skin incision there and excise a small amount of subcutaneous tissue, so that the knot can be buried and remain flat. There is no need to close this small incision. Postoperative dressing is unnecessary. Topical antibiotic ointment is applied for the skin wound.

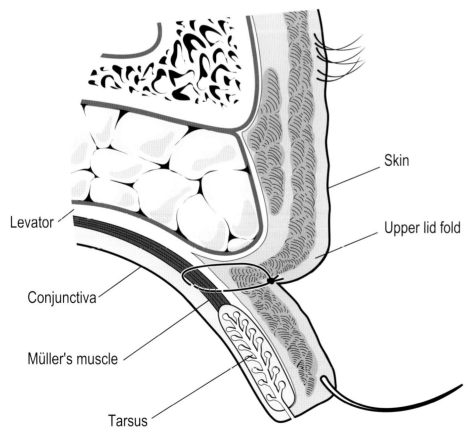

Fig. 18-7 Cross-sectional drawing showing the suture sling encompassing the subcutaneous tissues, orbicularis, levator aponeurosis, and Müller's muscle. Boo-Chai further commented that although this technique looks simple, it is technically difficult to execute unless one is experienced. The postoperative period is brief and the patient can go back to work after several days. The only drawback is that it is not always easy to obtain an equal crease width on both lids. The crease can be revised by removing the previously placed nylon slings and reapplying them at the desired level to correct any asymmetry.

References

1. Boo-Chai K. Further experience with cosmetic surgery of the upper eyelid. Proceedings of the Third International Congress of Plastic Surgery. Excerpta Medica International Congress Series No.66:518–524,1963.
2. Boo-Chai K. Secondary blepharoplasty in Orientals. In: Khoo B-C. Problems in plastic and reconstructive surgery. Vol.1. Philadelphia: JB Lippincott, 1991; 520–535.
3. Boo-Chai K. Perioperative bleeding in the pretarsal (post-aponeurotic) space in oriental blepharoplasty. Br J Plast Surg 2001;54:370.
4. Kim BG, Youn DY, Yoon ES et al. Unexpected bleeding caused by arterial variation inferolateral to levator palpebrae. Aesth Plast Surg 2003;27:123–125.
5. Kawai K, Imanishi N, Nakajima H et al. Arterial anatomic features of the upper palpebra. Plast Reconstruct Surg 2004;113:479–484.

Further Reading

1. Boo-Chai K. Further experience with cosmetic surgery of the upper eyelid. In: Broadbent TR, ed. Transactions of the Third International Congress of Plastic Surgery. Amsterdam: Excerpta Medica, 1964:518–524.
2. Boo-Chai K. Some aspects of plastic (cosmetic) surgery in Orientals. Br J Plast Surg 1969;22: 60–69.
3. Boo-Chai K. Aesthetic surgery for the Oriental. In: Barron JN, Saad MN, eds. Operative plastic and reconstructive surgery. Vol. 2. Edinburgh: Churchill Livingstone, 1980:761–781.
4. Boo-Chai K. Surgery for the oriental eyelid. In: Lewis JR Jr, ed. The art of aesthetic plastic surgery. Boston: Little, Brown, 1989: 611–617.
5. Boo-Chai K. The surgical anatomy of the oriental upper lid. World Plast 1996;1:230–236.

Park Z-epicanthoplasty

Jung Park

One of the anatomic characteristics found in many East Asian eyelids is the absence of a supratarsal crease, which allows the lax eyelid skin above the crease to descend and cover the tarsal margin and the eyelashes, and the concurrent presence of a medially positioned epicanthal fold. The net result is that the eyes appear smaller than they are owing to the apparent decrease in vertical height and horizontal length. The eyelashes also look much shorter than their actual length.

The medial canthal area shows distinctive anatomic variations owing to the presence or absence of the epicanthal folds. The epicanthal fold is a skin flap on the medial aspect of the eyelid covering the lacrimal lake in the medial canthal fornix. It descends over the lacrimal lake to attach the medial aspect of the lower eyelid. The epicanthal fold can be seen in 100% of both Asians and non-Asian group during 3–6 months of gestation. Beyond this period, during the second half of gestation, it disappears to a varying degree such that it is seen in only 2–5% of non-Asians in the general population, whereas in the Asian population the incidence of the epicanthal fold ranges between 40 and 90%, depending on the statistics.[1,2] The eyelid without the epicanthal fold is classified as type I. Type II is where the epicanthal fold partially covers the lacrimal lake and the fold ends at the margin of the lake. In type III, the lacrimal lake is covered almost completely by the epicanthal fold and the fold curves laterally to blend in with the lower eyelid. Type IV is a rare anomaly of reversed epicanthal fold. Types II and III are commonly encountered in Asian blepharoplasty.

When the upper eyelid skin is still relaxed and hanging over the eyelashes, the skin of the medial canthal fold is also relaxed. The natural epicanthal fold curves smoothly from the medial canthus to the rest of the eyelid. As the pretarsal upper eyelid skin is drawn up higher following the double-eyelid surgery, the skin of the epicanthal fold becomes stretched tight. This tightening of the normally relaxed epicanthal fold creates a sharp skin ridge similar to a web formation. The palpebral fissure may turns into an undesirable round eye, with a somewhat startling appearance. Epican-thoplasty can enhance the aesthetic result of double-eyelid surgery by lengthening the palpebral fissure, thereby producing the image of a larger and more open eye. A long parallel fold starting from the nasal end to the lateral canthal end brings out the natural beauty of the eye.

Despite many procedures available to eliminate the epicanthal fold, many surgeons are reluctant to perform epicanthoplasty for fear of creating a visible scar in the medial canthal area. Even a minor scar is not tolerated in this area. Problems associated with the various epicanthoplasty designs are complex incisions extending beyond the eyelid skin, and tension across the suture line generated by pulling the tissue to advance the flap. The purpose of many classic papers on epicantho-plasty was the correction of congenital anomalies or a traumatic epicanthal web, where minor scarring is not as critically scrutinized. My experience with previously described procedures has been unsatisfactory as a result of:

1. Complex incisions running in diverse directions.
2. Inability to incorporate the medial canthal incisions with the rest of the incision for the double-eyelid procedure
3. Lack of clear landmarks and reference points in design.

The skin in the medial canthal area is quite restricted in width and blends rapidly into the adjacent thick nasal skin. The beauty of the Z-epicanthoplasty is that the incisions are within the thin eyelid skin, can be incorporated into the incision for the double-eyelid procedure, and the technique provides for a tension-free closure.[3-5] The design follows clear fixed landmarks and reference points, such as the medial margin of the lacrimal lake, the incision line for the double-eyelid procedure, and the fusion point between the epicanthal fold and the lower eyelid skin. The design is simple, easy to understand and reproduce. It leaves minimal and clean scars. It is unlikely to involve the nasal skin. Following Z-epicanthoplasty, the double-eyelid folds become parallel to the eyelid margin for a

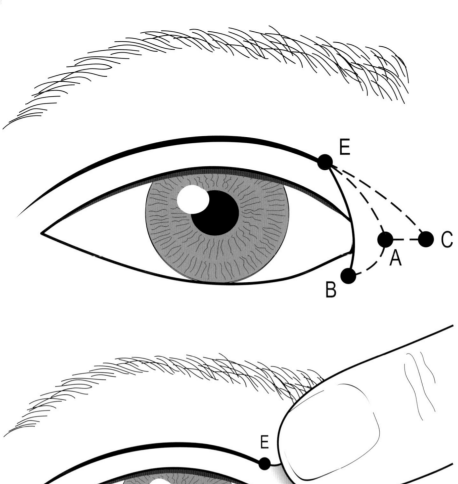

Fig. 19-1 Marking for Z-epicanthoplasty incision. Point A is marked as a surface representation of point D at the medial end of the lacrimal lake. The marking for the double-eyelid incision is also seen.

Fig. 19-2 Line D–B. A short line is drawn to connect point B, the confluence of the epicanthal fold, with the lower eyelid skin. The epicanthal fold is retracted to show point D. The line D–B is visible. The marking for the double-eyelid incision is extended to point A. This line gently converges towards the tarsal margin.

parallel crease as they approach the medial canthal area, and gradually fade away.

In spite of the sound concept, the execution of the procedure is highly dependent on surgical technique. The benefit of having a widely open eye with a long and beautiful parallel double-eyelid fold versus the risk of possible redness and a visible scar should be thoroughly discussed with the patient. Although this procedure leaves a minimal scar when it is performed exactly as designed, some patients may not tolerate even the slightest scar.

Procedure

Surgery is performed in the office under local anesthesia with oral sedation. Markings for the incision are made

in the holding area using a fine felt-tip marker while the patient is in a sitting position with the eyes in the primary gaze position. The patient is instructed to open or close the eyes, depending on the area of marking. The first marking is for the incision to create the double-eyelid fold, if needed. Next, a point is marked on the surface of the epicanthal fold as a surface representation of the medial-most point of the lacrimal lake. This is designated point A (Fig. 19-1). Point B is the point of confluence of the epicanthal fold with the lower eyelid skin, and is quite distinctive in most patients. Point D is the medial-most end of the lacrimal lake (Fig. 19-2). When points A and D are viewed from the front through a transparent layer of the epicanthal fold, A and D should be the same point. Thus, the lines A–B and D–B should be equal in length and should be the same line

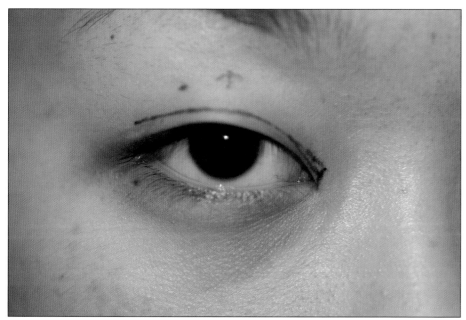

Fig. 19-3 The second line is drawn parallel to the tarsal margin. Point E is where the two lines diverge from the double-eyelid marking. A line is drawn obliquely from point A. The cross point between these two lines is point C. A small triangle is created. This triangle will be removed later.

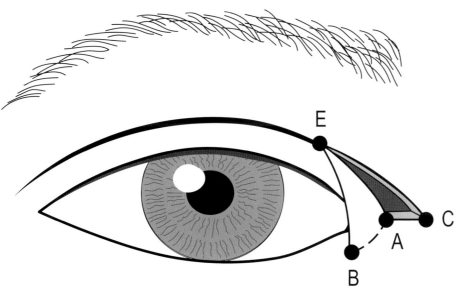

Fig. 19-4 Removal of triangle EAC. When the eyelid skin is removed in double-eyelid operation, the upper incision runs parallel to the tarsal margins. The EAC triangle is then incorporated into the eyelid skin excision.

when viewed from the front. The incisions A–B and D–B should close without any tension. Point E is on the line drawn for the double-eyelid incision. While the patient is in a primary gaze position, marking for the double-eyelid procedure is extended medially, aiming at point A. The line shows a slight tendency to converge towards the tarsal margin. Next, a second line is drawn as a medial continuation of the double-eyelid incision. This time the line maintains a parallel relationship with the tarsal margin (Fig. 19-3). Next, a line is drawn from point A horizontally or angled superomedially to join the upper line. The cross point becomes point C. Point E is where the two lines diverge from the main

double-eyelid incision to meet point A and point C, respectively.

In modified Z-epicanthoplasty the angled line A–C maintains point C closer to the eyelid and seems to achieve a better parallel relationship. Line A–C can be up to 45° from the horizontal. When excision of a strip of skin is indicated for the double-eyelid operation, the triangle EAC is incorporated with the pretarsal eyelid skin strip (Fig. 19-4). In a patient with double eyelids Z-epicanthoplasty markings are made by placing point E on the supratarsal crease.

Local anesthetic is infiltrated after marking to avoid distortion. Efforts should be made to avoid wetting the

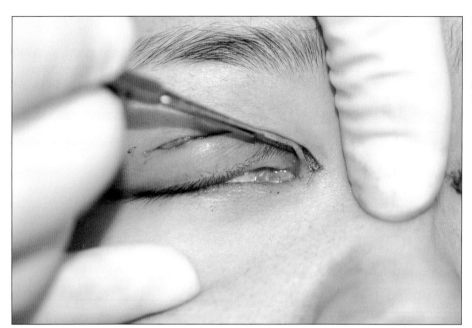

Fig. 19-5 Point D, the medial end of the lacrimal lake, is identified. A no. 15 Bard–Parker blade is inserted with the blade up and facing the surgeon. The tip of the blade touches the medial canthal ligament.

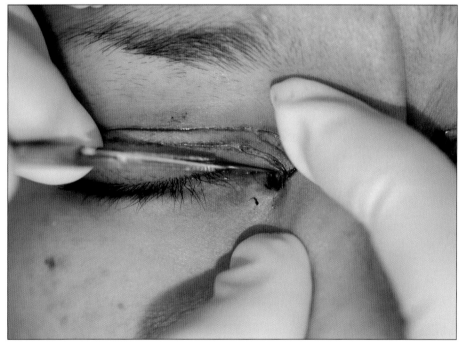

Fig. 19-6 The surgeon pushes the blade gently but forcefully, following line D–B.

incision with the anesthetic solution. Surgery without an exact design guarantees a closure with tension and a thick scar. Supplemental local anesthetic should be injected deep into the surface of the medial canthal ligament, as this is one area where the patient often experiences pain if not adequately injected.

I start the incision for the Z-epicanthoplasty before the incision for the double eyelid because of the need for precision in this small and critical area. The skin of the triangle EAC or a pretarsal skin strip is excised and discarded (Fig. 19-4). The EAB incision is made deep through the muscle, reaching the medial canthal ligament. The incision D–B should be a straight line. A no.15 Bard–Parker blade is inserted with the blade up and facing the surgeon. The tip of the blade touches the medial canthus immediately above the conjunctiva. While the assistant is spreading the epicanthal fold flat with the fingers, the surgeon pushes the blade gently but forcefully following the line D–B (Figs 19-5,19-6). A curvilinear incision on the lower eyelid skin laterally

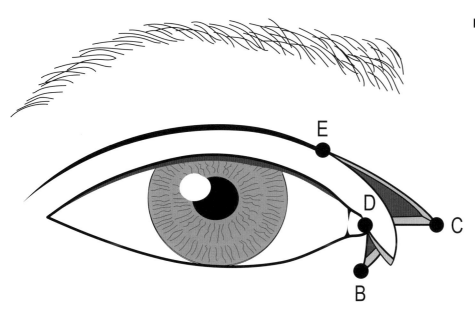

Fig. 19-7 Elevation of flap EABD.

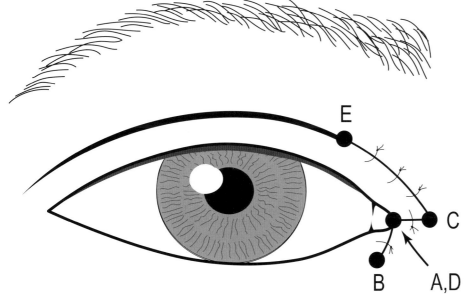

Fig. 19-8 Closure. Points A and D are sutured together.

will create a gap in closure between lines A–B and D–B, which causes tension across the suture line. The flap EABD is then grasped and lifted up tight at point B with atraumatic forceps. The remaining adherence of the flap to the medial canthal ligament is then severed with the knife in a pushing and sweeping motion over the surface of the ligament. A pair of sharp-pointed tenotomy scissors may be used for this purpose. The surgeon will feel a sudden release of the flap from the ligament. This step is one of the most important aspects of the dissection in order to ensure a tension-free flap rotation and closure (Fig. 19-7). Once this is accomplished, the rotated

flap will fill the recipient triangle EAC (Fig. 19-8), completely relaxed and with no gaping of the line E–C (Figs 19-9, 19-10, 19-11). Because the flap is free of tension, a deep fixation suture to keep it in place is not necessary. The incision lines DA–B and DA–C eventually fade (Fig. 19-12). If the surgeon desires a more distinctive medial crease, the incision E–C is undermined toward the orbital portion of the upper eyelid, and an anchoring suture can be placed between the rotated EAB flap and the deep soft tissue at the orbital side under the incision E–C. A 6/0 or 7/0 clear nylon suture is used with buried knots. Every effort should be made

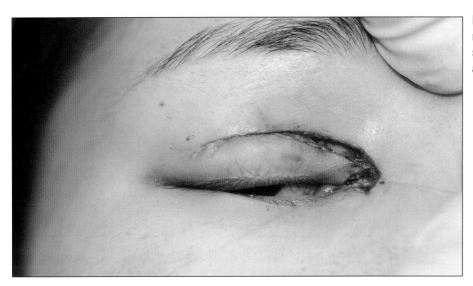

Fig. 19-9 The flap is rotated and maintains its position without the aid of sutures. The skin adjacent to points A and D is sutured together.

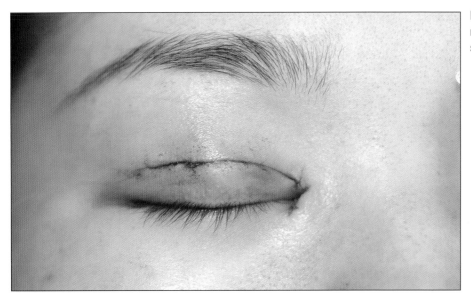

Fig. 19-10 The flap maintains the rotated position without tension. No suture is placed for the flap.

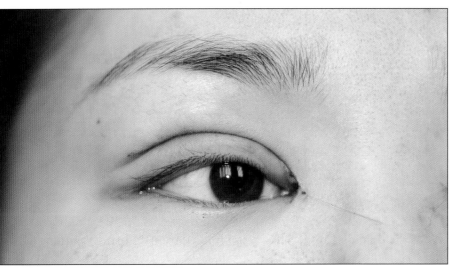

Fig. 19-11 The flap in position with the eyes open and without suture fixation.

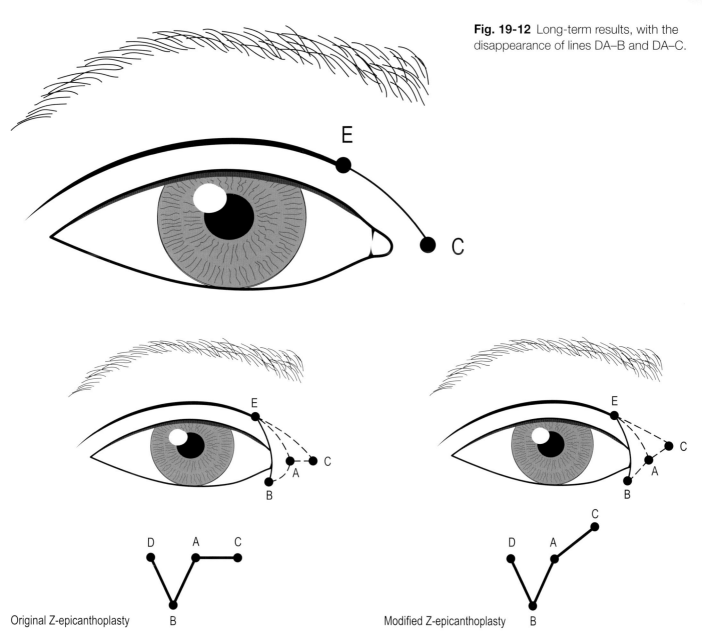

Fig. 19-12 Long-term results, with the disappearance of lines DA–B and DA–C.

Original Z-epicanthoplasty

Modified Z-epicanthoplasty

Fig. 19-13 The original Z-epicanthoplasty and the modified Z-epicanthoplasty.

to avoid placing the suture superficially, otherwise it may create prolonged redness and, at times, even granuloma formation. If the epicanthal fold is excessively large, the edge of the flap along EAB may be trimmed conservatively. Suturing between points D and A is at times a technical challenge. If it is not easy, or if the suture needle cuts through the ligament, then the suture may be passed through the eyelid skin close to points D and A. For patients with abundant fat in the medial canthal area, defatting under the incision A–B is neces-

sary to match the thinness of the line D–B, which has very little soft tissue at point D. Otherwise, a step formation develops at the closure site. The skin is closed with 6/0 fast-absorbing gut sutures. The angle ECA is about 45° in the original Z-epicanthoplasty with a horizontal A–C, and up to 90° in the modified Z-epicanthoplasty having an oblique A–C. Both the original and the modified Z-epicanthoplasty result in a distinctively different closure pattern (Fig. 19-13).

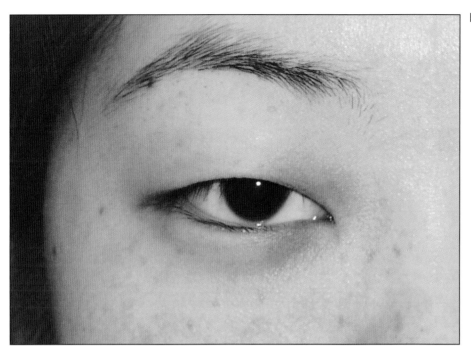

Fig. 19-14 Pre-Z-epicanthoplasty.

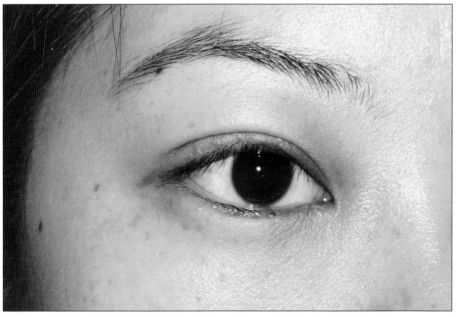

Fig. 19-15 Same patient as in Figure 19-13, 1 year after double-eyelid operation and Z-epicanthoplasty.

Scar formation is the most critical issue associated with epicanthoplasty. The common causes of unsightly scar formation are poor design and closure with tension. One critical issue is to determine point A in a more conservative location laterally, closer to the eye than to the nose. When point A is marked more medially and further from point D than it should be, point A has to be stretched laterally to meet point D during closure, which will create tension on the closure and result in a thicker scar.[6,7] Exact placement of point A and complete detachment of the flap at point D are two critical steps of the operation. Extremely conservative excision of triangle EAC is also an important aspect in preventing scar formation. Figures 19-14 and 19-15 illustrate pre and post operative appearance following double-eyelid operation and Z-epicanthoplasty.

Complications

Complications are related to the sutures and to scar formation. The medial canthal skin tolerates suture materials poorly owing to the delicate nature of the skin. Any permanent fixation suture should be placed deep to the orbicularis muscle. Even then, the suture material may migrate to the surface, causing redness and/or granuloma formation. It is better to free the epicanthal flap completely and avoid the use of anchoring sutures. A step formation at the closure line of A–B and D–B creates an annoying visible scar. This tiny scar on the medial part of the lower eyelid at the medial canthal area often gives an appearance of a foreign body. This problem is avoided by leveling the skin surface between lines A–B and D–B. At times defatting under line A–B is required to match the thin line D–B. Hypertrophic scarring is due to tension in the closure. The patient should be carefully screened for the possibility of keloid formation. Small doses of steroid injection may alleviate thick scars and keloid.

References

1. Liu D, Hsu WM. Oriental eyelids: anatomic difference and surgical consideration. Ophthalmol Plast Reconstruct Surg 1986;2:59–64.
2. Ohmori K. Aesthetic surgery in Asian eyelids. In: McCarthy JG. Plastic surgery. Vol 3. Philadelphia: WB Saunders, 1990: 2415–2435.
3. Park JI. Z-epicanthoplasty in Asian eyelids. Plast Reconstruct Surg 1996;98:602.
4. Park JI. Modified Z-epicanthoplasty in the Asian eyelid. Arch Facial Plast Surg 2000;2:43.
5. Park JI. Park Z-epicanthoplasty. In: Park JI, Toriumi D. Cosmetic surgery for the Asian face. Philadelphia: WB Saunders, [to be published].
6. Yoo WM, Park SH, Kwag DR. Root Z-epicanthoplasty in Asian eyelids. Plast Reconstruct Surg 2002;109:2067.
7. Park JI. Root Z-epicanthoplasty in Asian eyelids. Correspondence and brief communications. Plast Reconstruct Surg 2003;111:2477.

Outlook – Challenges in Aesthetic Surgery of the Asian Eyelid

Chapter 20

William P.D. Chen

The Challenge of Aesthetic Surgery on the Asian Eyelid

The most important point in the plethora of techniques available for the construction of an upper eyelid crease in Asians is that the external incision methods are an attempt to produce surgical adhesions between the distal fibers of the levator aponeurosis (or superior tarsal border) and the skin, inferior subcutaneous plane, or pretarsal platform. The myriad variants of the suture ligation techniques try to produce a tight tissue plane between the distal portion of the levator aponeurosis (or the upper portion of the tarsus) and the pretarsal tissues inferior and anterior to the aponeurosis, whether they be subcutaneous tissues or pretarsal orbicularis muscle, or to eliminate dead space between pretarsal skin and tarsus. In both the external incision and the suture ligation methods, a firm pretarsal platform is linked to the levator aponeurosis. This platform telescopes superiorly at its junction with the supratarsal skin to form the upper lid crease.

The Challenges

When progressing from preoperative planning to the actual surgical stages of an Asian blepharoplasty, the surgeon must shift from a two-dimensional mode of thinking with a clear concept of crease placement to a three-dimensional mode to approach the layers of the upper eyelids. I prefer to think of the progression from one end of the eyelid to the other as traveling through many different terrains. To digress with an analogy, the Great Wall of China is the only manmade structure that can be seen from space by orbiting astronauts. At ground level, it traverses through vastly different terrains and climate patterns, although the basic structures of its throughways, fortresses, and storage garrisons may appear similar they are not. The challenge in working on the eyelid is to construct a functional and continuous structure even though it

passes through different areas with different topographic features.

Each vertical section of the eyelid is composed of a different subset of tissues of varying sizes and thicknesses. For example, the vertical height of the tarsus is shorter over the medial and lateral extents; there is more pretarsal fat over the central portion of the eyelid; the levator aponeurotic attachment over the medial and lateral horns is thin and less vertically oriented; the medial upper lid fold may interfere with crease formation; the lacrimal gland may interfere with lateral crease placement; the upper lid dermis laterally is thicker and less likely to invaginate when one attempts to make a crease; and the central presence of the preaponeurotic fat pads can obliterate an otherwise well positioned and well formed crease.

The challenge is to produce a crease that is continuous and aesthetically pleasing as it traverses the different terrains of the upper lid. In each section of the upper lid, factors that can interfere with the optimal formation of a dynamic crease have to be eliminated. The result should be a crease that provides optimal height, shape, continuity, and permanence.

A Look to the Future

Progress in the development of this frequently performed Asian cosmetic operation has been quite steady from 1896 to the present. The early Japanese medical literature blazed the trail for the subsequent modifications of both the ligation techniques and the external incision methods used in the east and the west. The future looks bright for the continuing evolution of Asian blepharoplasty.

I anticipate the availability of better suture materials, perhaps made of polymers that are fully nonreactive and tissue compatible. Used in either the incision or ligation methods, such materials, especially if they can be made to last 3–12 months before dissolving, would reduce the incidence of suboptimal results and allow more creativity in technique; biocompatible polymers could be designed to be implanted within the eyelid. For example, implanting a thin shield in the pretarsal plane could result in adhesions between the pretarsal orbicularis muscle and the overlying skin and produce a firm pretarsal platform without causing noticeable scarring. Biocompatible polymers or composite alloys may be engineered into microclips or tacks, such that several could be implanted along the superior tarsal border as an expansion or extension of the distal fibers of the levator aponeurosis. Lasers using elements other than argon, yttrium–aluminum–garnet (YAG), or potassium titanyl-phosphate (KTP-YAG), may be available in the future and could be used to produce controlled aponeurotic adhesions, simulating the physiologic adhesions and interdigitations seen in eyelids that have natural creases.

I see further research and analysis on the dynamics of the eyelid crease, perhaps using currently available real-time tools such as the PET scan, or yet to be invented nano-devices, studying the levator aponeurosis, tarsus, and preaponeurotic tissues (tarsoligamentous junction). There will be continued innovation in new suture materials and synthetic implants that can be used to facilitate lid crease formation. Suborbicularis thermoplastic cauterization using microvoltage current on a needle tip, and radiofrequency cold needles in cautery mode have already been tried.

Look for future trends: minimally invasive means of excision of tissue redundancy using endoscopic principles; central partial incision with fat debulking coupled with medial and lateral suborbicularis cautery; as well as buried ligatures delivered through different avenues.

I wish you well in your continued journey for perfection in this type of aesthetic surgery.

Pre-1952 Japanese Literature on Cosmetic Eyelid Surgery (in Japanese)

Pre-1952 Japanese Literature on Cosmetic Eyelid Surgery (in Japanese)				
Author	K Mikamo	K Uchida	M Maruo	B Hata
Year	1896	1926	1929	1933
Journal	J Chugaishinpo	Jpn J Ophthalmol 30(5):593	Jpn Rev Clin Ophthalmol 24:393–405	Jpn Rev Clin Ophthalmol 28:491–494
Country	Japan	Japan	Japan	Japan
Crease height	6–8 mm	7–8 mm fan shape (semilunar)	7 mm	10 mm
Suture method	Yes	Yes		Yes
Incision method			Incise skin	
Remove skin	No	No	No	
Orbicularis			Sub Q dissection superiorly and inferiorly to incision	
Orbital septum				
Preaponeurotic fat				
Crease formed by	3 trans-lid sutures from conjunctiva to skin	3 trans-lid sutures, ligate 2 mm tissue horizontally	4 throws with single 5-0 catgut suture	3 trans-lid sutures
Suture	4-0 silk	Buried catgut	Catgut suture skin/tarsus/skin	5-0 silk through tarsus to skin; tied down with beads
Days left in	2–6	4		8–10
Variations	Depth of crease related to days sutures left in		Alternatively, trans-lid suture from conjunctiva above STB to anterior skin surface	

continued

Pre-1952 Japanese Literature on Cosmetic Eyelid Surgery (in Japanese)				
Author	K Hayashi	K Hayashi	S Inoue	Y Mitsui
Year	1938	1938	1947	1950
Journal	*Jpn Rev Clin Ophthalmol* 33:1000–1010	*Jpn Rev Clin Ophthalmol* 33:1098–1110	*Jpn Rev Clin Ophthalmol* 27(11):306	*Jpn Rev Clin Ophthalmol* 44:19
Country	Japan	Japan	Japan	Japan
Crease height	Medially 5; centrally 6; laterally 7. Creates medially tapered crease			
Suture method	Yes			
Incision method		Yes	Yes	Yes
Remove skin				
Orbicularis		Excision of pretarsal orbicularis	Dissection of subcutaneous connective tissue between crease incision line and eyelid margin	Removes pretarsal orbicularis, and fat
Orbital septum				
Preaponeurotic fat				
Crease formed by	Central and lateral stitches above crease; medial stitch below crease line and passes through tarsus	Interrupted skin/tarsus/skin closure, plus in-between skin/skin stitch	Skin/tarsus/skin	Five 5-0 nylon sutures: Inferior skin edge to tarsus (2–3 days) Skin/skin closure with 5-0 silk
Suture		4-0 silk	5-0 silk	
Days left in		4	2–3	7–8
Variations				

continued

Pre-1952 Japanese Literature on Cosmetic Eyelid Surgery (in Japanese)		
Author	K Hirose	K Ohashi	T Ikegami
Year	1950	1951	1951
Journal	*Jpn Rev Clin Ophthalmol* 45:374	*Jpn Rev Clin Ophthalmol* 46:723	*Jpn Rev Clin Ophthalmol* 46:706–708
Country	Japan	Japan	Japan
Crease height			
Suture method		Cautery method	
Incision method	Yes		Yes
Remove skin			
Orbicularis			
Orbital septum			
Preaponeurotic fat			
Crease formed by		Electrocoagulation needle; 7 burns along the crease line and 2 rows of burns below it	
Suture			
Days left in			
Variations			

Modern Literature on Asian Eyelid Surgery (in English)

Modern Literature on Asian Eyelid Surgery (in English)			
Author	BT Sayoc	DR Millard	LR Fernandez	LR Fernandez
Year	1954	1955	1960	1960
Journal	*Am J Ophthalmol* 38(4):556–559	*Plast Reconstruct Surg* 16(5):319–336	*Plast Reconstruct Surg* 25:257–264	*Plast Reconstruct Surg* 25:257–264
Country	Phillippines	USA/Korea	USA/Hawaii	USA/Hawaii
Conjunctival suturing				
Skin incision	Yes		Simple	Radical
Remove skin		3 mm	7–8 mm	8–10 mm
Orbicularis	1–3 mm orbicularis	Trim inferior edge		3–5 mm orbicularis
Orbital septum		Open	Open	3–5 mm
Preaponeurotic fat		Lipectomy		Excised fat
Crease form	Inf. skin/tarsus	Skin to tarsus	Inf. skin/levator	Inf. subcut. tissue/levator
Suture	Buried 6-0 silk or chromic catgut	Interrupted silk	3 buried 5-0 nylon	3 5-0 nylon and 6-0 nylon
Days left in	5		For skin sutures, 3	3
Effectiveness	'Static' crease		Superficial	Deep, permanent
Comments	Related articles published in *AJO* 1956;41: 1040 *AJO* 1956;42:298 *AJO* 1961;52:122 *AJO* 1967;63:155 Included fat excision *Clinics in Plast Surg* 1974;1:157	See also *Am J Ophthalmol* 1964;57:646	'Dynamic'	'Dynamic'

continued

Modern Literature on Asian Eyelid Surgery (in English)				
Author	HG Pang	J Uchida	Khoo Boo-Chai	Khoo Boo-Chai
Year	1961	1962	1963	1969
Journal	*Arch Ophthalmol* 65:783–784	*Br J Plast Surg* 18:271–276	*Plast Reconstruct Surg* 31:74–78	*Br J Plast Surg* 22(1):60–69
Country	USA/Hawaii	Japan	Malaysia/Singapore	Singapore
Conjunctival suturing				Yes (3)
Skin incision		Yes	Yes	3 nicks
Remove skin			Sometimes	
Orbicularis		Thins pretarsal orbicularis	Thins pretarsal orbicularis	
Orbital septum		Open	Open	
Preaponeurotic fat		Trim some fat	Removes some fat	
Crease form	Double-armed suture, from skin to conjunctiva to skin	Tarsus/inf. skin	Skin/tarsus/skin	
Suture	Three 4-0 silk	Three 2-0 chromic	Silk	6-0 silk
Days left in	10	Remove in 3	10	
Effectiveness	May disappear			
Comments		Discussed pretarsal, subcutaneous, submuscular, and orbital fat	Skin/levator/skin method discussed in Barron JN, Saad MN, eds. Operative plastic and reconstructive surgery. Edinburgh: Churchill Livingstone, 1980:761–781.	Mostly a discussion on trends of plastic surgery in Asians. Also discussed skin incision and excision of skin, orbicularis muscle, and fat.

continued

Modern Literature on Asian Eyelid Surgery (in English)				
Author	S Ohmori	Y Mutou, H Mutou	JH Sheen	CZ Weingarten
Year	1972	1972	1974	1976
Journal	Ch. 19. Transformation of the Oriental eye into the Western eye. In Goldwyn RM (Ed.): The Unfavourable Results in Plastic Surgery: Avoidance and Treatment 1972: 275–282. Boston: Little, Brown	*Br J Plast Surg* 25(3):285–291	*Plast Reconstruct Surg* 54(4):424–431	*Trans Am Acad Ophthalmol Otolaryngol* 82:442–446
Country	Japan	Japan	USA	USA/Thailand
Conjunctival suturing		Yes (2)		
Skin incision	Yes		Yes	Yes
Remove skin	Sometimes		Yes	Variable
Orbicularis	Thins pretarsal orbicularis		Remove orbicularis	Trim inferior edge
Orbital septum	Thins submuscular fat		Open	Open
Preaponeurotic fat	Remove variable amounts of preaponeurotic fat		Excised	Excised
Crease form	Conjunctiva to skin		Levator/inf. orbic.	STB/inf. subcut. tissue
Suture	3-0 chromic catgut and 6-0 nylon	Buried 6-0 nylon or synthetic catgut	Buried 7-0 silk	Buried 6-0 chromic
Days left in	3		Routine closure	
Effectiveness			Crease is not obvious with eyelids closed	
Comments			Also described tarsus-to-orbicularis and tarsus-to-skin closure	Surgery performed on Thai patients

continued

Modern Literature on Asian Eyelid Surgery (in English)			
Author	AM Putterman, MJ Urist	R Rubenzik	Y Hiraga	JS Zubiri
Year	1976	1977	1980	1981
Journal	*Arch Ophthalmol* 94(11):1941–1954	*Ann Ophthalmol* 9(9):1189–1192	*Clinics in Plast Surg* 7(4):553–567	*Clinics in Plast Surg* 8(4):725–737
Country	USA	USA	Japan	Philippines
Conjunctival suturing				
Skin incision	Yes	Yes	Yes	Yes
Remove skin				Yes
Orbicularis		Trim inferior edge	Trim orbicularis	2–3 mm
Orbital septum		Open	Open	Excise 2 mm
Preaponeurotic fat		Excised	Excised	Excised
Crease form	STB/inf. subcut. tissue	Skin/lev./skin	Skin/lev./skin	Skin/STB/levator
Suture	Buried 6-0 polyester plus Pang's 6-0 silk	6-0 nylon or silk	Nylon	Buried 6-0 nylon, plus skin 6-0 nylon
Days left in		5		6
Effectiveness				
Comments				

continued

Modern Literature on Asian Eyelid Surgery (in English)				
Author	LC Hin	KC Chua	JA McCurdy	T Onizuka, M Iwanami
Year	1981	1982	1982	1984
Journal	*Ann Plast Surg* 7(5):362–374	*Aesthetic Plast Surg* 6(4):221–223	*Otolaryngol Head Neck Surg* 90(1):142–145	*Aesthetic Plast Surg* 8(2):97–100
Country	Singapore	Singapore	USA	Japan
Conjunctival suturing				
Skin incision	Yes	Yes	Yes	
Remove skin	Yes	Variable	Yes	
Orbicularis			3–5 mm	
Orbital septum	Open		Open	
Preaponeurotic fat		Excised	Variable	
Crease form	Skin/levator/skin	Levator/inf. subcut. tissue	Skin/levator/skin	
Suture	5-0 silk	Buried 6-0 polyglycolic sutures; skin closure: 6-0 nylon	6-0 nylon (7 days); 6-0 nylon subQ (3 days)	
Days left in	5	5		
Effectiveness				
Comments	See also *Ann Plast Surg* 1985;14(6): 523–534			Discussion of why people prefer double eyelids

continued

Modern Literature on Asian Eyelid Surgery (in English)				
Author	Y Shirakabe, et al	RS Matsunaga	RY Song	WPD Chen
Year	1985	1985	1985	1987
Journal	*Ann Plast Surg* 15(3):224–241	*Arch Otolaryngol* 111(3):149–153	*Aesthetic Plast Surg* 9(3):173–180	*Ophthal Plast Reconstr Surg* 3(3):135–140
Country	Japan	USA	China	USA
Conjunctival suturing				
Skin incision	Yes	Yes	3 small incisions	Yes
Remove skin	No			Variable
Orbicularis	Undermine pretarsal connective tissue	Trim pretarsal orbicularis muscle and fat		2–3 mm
Orbital septum				Open
Preaponeurotic fat		Variable		Variable
Crease form	Translid suturing with 6 double-armed sutures tied with beads	Skin/STB/skin	Tarsus/subcut. tissue	Skin/levator/skin
Suture	6-0 nylon	Buried 6-0 polyglycolic acid sutures	Buried 6-0 nylon	6-0 and 7-0 nylon or silk
Days left in	8			5 to 7
Effectiveness				
Comments	Gave account of Japanese techniques: 1896 Mikamo 1912 Onishi 1926 Uchida 1926 Nakamura 1927 Kitajima 1929 Maruo* 1933 Hata 1938 K. Hayashi* 1947 Inoue* 1949 Hirai* 1950 Mazume 1950 Mitsui* 1950 M. Hayashi 1950 Takano 1950 Ohashi 1951 Hirose* 1951 Hirai* 1951 Ikegami* 1950 Momo (* = incision)			First coined the term *Asian blepharoplasty*; discussed crease shapes and technique

continued

Modern Literature on Asian Eyelid Surgery (in English)				
Author	PY Yang	KY Song	SM Baek	EJ Weng
Year	1987	1988	1989	1989
Journal	*Chin J Plast Surg Burn* 3(3):191–192	*Chin J Plast Surg Burn* 4(1):6–9	*Plast Reconstruct Surg* 83(2):236–243	*Plast Reconstruct Surg* 83(4):622–628
Country	China	China	Korea	Taiwan
Conjunctival suturing			Ligature technique	
Skin incision			2 stab incisions in skin; single stitch	Yes
Remove skin	Puncture with threaded needle then tunnel under orbicularis and levator aponeurosis			
Orbicularis				
Orbital septum				
Preaponeurotic fat				
Crease form	Skin/tarsus/skin continuous or reverse looping		Single stitch encompasses subconj./levator/ subcut. tissues	Levator/inf. subcut. tissue
Suture	4-0 silk; compress with rubber catheter		Buried 6-0 polypropylene (Prolene) sutures	Buried 6-0 polypropylene (Prolene) sutures
Days left in	7			
Effectiveness			Crease disappeared in 2.9% of cases per author	
Comments	"Twisted needle" may elicit hematoma	A general discussion of concepts of beauty and double eyelid		Discussed complications of oriental blepharoplasty

continued

Modern Literature on Asian Eyelid Surgery (in English)			
Author	KY Song	YH Bang	WPD Chen
Year	1990	1991	1994
Journal	*Chin J Plast Surg* 6:96–97	*Plast Reconstruct Surg* 88:12–17	*Asian Blepharoplasty (A Surgical Atlas)* Butterworth-Heinemann (First Edition)
Country	China	Korea	USA
Conjunctival suturing			
Skin incision	3 stab incisions	Yes	
Remove skin		No	
Orbicularis		Trims orbicularis muscle, connective tissue, and pretarsal fat	
Orbital septum			
Preaponeurotic fat		Remove fat if prolapsed inferiorly	
Crease form	Transcutaneous intratarsal and intradermal suturing	Skin to orbicularis: basting sutures	
Suture	3 buried stitches	3 6-0 silk	
Days left in		5 to 6	
Effectiveness			
Comments			First textbook on this topic: Detailed terminology, cultural perception, comparitive anatomy, crease variation, shape, height, continuity and permanence; main schools of technique, complications, revisions and literature publications

continued

Modern Literature on Asian Eyelid Surgery (in English)			
Author	Li Dong et al	WPD Chen	JI Park	JS Lee, WJ Park, MS Shin, IC Song
Year	1994	1996	1996	1997
Journal	*Chin J Plast Surg Burns* 10:436, *Plast Reconstruct Surg* 1996;98(5):919	*Plast Reconstruct Surg* 97(1):212–218 Triangular, Trapezoidal and Rectangular debulking of Eyelid tissues in Asian Blepharoplasty	*Plast Reconstruct Surg* 98(4):602–609 Z-epicanthoplasty	*Plast Reconstruct Surg* 100(1):170–178 'Septodermal' Fixation Technique
Country	China (Beijing Med Univ)	USA	USA	Korea (Samsung Med Center)
Conjunctival suturing				
Skin incision		Yes	Yes	Variable placement of skin/septum-levator attachment
Remove skin		Yes	By flap transposition	
Orbicularis		Trims orbicularis		
Orbital septum		Opens septum		
Preaponeurotic fat		Variable		
Crease form		Skin/apon./skin		
Suture		6-0 interrupted sutures and 7-0 continuous suture		
Days left in		5–7 days		
Effectiveness		Permanent		
Comments	Emphasizes removal of fascial tissues in double blepharoplasty (review by Boo-Chai in Int Abstracts of PRS)		*Arch Facial Plast Surg* 2000;2(10):43–47 Modified Z-Epicanthoplasty	

continued

Modern Literature on Asian Eyelid Surgery (in English)				
Author	Sergile, Obata	JW Kim, JO Lee	KC Yoon, S Park	YS Kao, CH Lin, RH Fang
Year	1997	1998	1998	1998
Journal	*Plast Reconstruct Surg* 99(3):662–667 translation of Mikamo's 1896 paper	*Aesth Plast Surg* 22(6):433–438 Asian Blepharoplasty with short-pulsed Contact ND-Yag Laser: limited incision	*Plast Reconstruct Surg* 102(2):502–508 Selective tissue removal in bleph for young Asians	*Plast Reconstruct Surg* 102(6): 1835–1841 Epicanthoplasty with Y-V advancement
Country	USA	Korea	Korea (U. of Ulsan)	Taiwan (Vet. Gen Hosp)
Conjunctival suturing				
Skin incision		Yes		
Remove skin		Yes		
Orbicularis		Yes		
Orbital septum		Yes		
Preaponeurotic fat		Yes		
Crease form		Levator/tarsus/skin		
Suture		7-0 nylon, or tissue glue		
Days left in				
Effectiveness				
Comments			A general discussion on incisional technique	

continued

Modern Literature on Asian Eyelid Surgery (in English)				
Author	JI Park	SL Jeong, BN Lemke, RK Dortzbach et al	YH Bang, HH Chu, SH Park et al	YW Kim, HJ Park, S Kim
Year	1999	1999	1999	2000
Journal	*Arch Facial Plast Surg* 1(2):90–95 Orbic-Levator Fixation	*Arch Ophthalmol* 117(7):907–912 Comparison of Asian & Cauc. Upper Lid Anatomy	*Plast Reconstruct Surg* 103(6):1788–1791 The Fallacy of the Levator Expansion Theory	*Plast Reconstruct Surg* 106(6): 1399–1404 Revisional correction by interposing preaponeurotic fat
Country	USA	Korea (Chonnam U), USA	Korea (Inha Gen Hosp)	Korea (Ewha Women Univ)
Conjunctival suturing				
Skin incision	Yes			
Remove skin	Yes			
Orbicularis				
Orbital septum	Opens			
Preaponeurotic fat				
Crease form	Orbic/levator			
Suture				
Days left in				
Effectiveness				
Comments				

continued

Modern Literature on Asian Eyelid Surgery (in English)				
Author	RS Sim, JD Smith, AS Chan	Y Lee, E Lee, WJ Park	DH Kang, SH Koo, JH Choi et al	Yang
Year	2000	2000	2001	2001
Journal	*Arch Facial Plast Surg* 2(2):113–120 Comparison of aesthetic facial proportions of Chinese & Caucasian women	*Plast Reconstruct Surg* 105(5):1872–1880 Anchor Epicanthoplasty combined with Outer-type lid crease procedure	*Plast Reconstruct Surg* 107(7): 1884–1889 Use of CO_2 laser	*Annals of Plast Surg* 46(4):364–368 Double Eyelid: A Limited Incision technique
Country	Singapore (National U)	Korea (Seoul National U)	Korea (Univ. MC)	Korea (Catholic U)
Conjunctival suturing				
Skin incision			Yes	4 mm skin incision
Remove skin			Yes	
Orbicularis				
Orbital septum			Opened	
Preaponeurotic fat			Optional	Optional removal
Crease form			6-0 vicryl: inferior skin to tarsus/levator	Levator/tarsus to skin/muscle
Suture				
Days left in				
Effectiveness				
Comments	General Aesthetics			

continued

Modern Literature on Asian Eyelid Surgery (in English)				
Author	J Cheng, FZ Xu	Miyake, Hiraga	MT Yen, DR Jordan, RL Anderson	BC Cho, KY Lee
Year	2001	2001	2002	2002
Journal	*Plast Reconstruct Surg* 107(7):1665–1668 Microstructure of asian eyelid crease	*Jpn J Plast Reconstruct Surg* 44:815 Selection of skin resection or double eyelid operation	*Ophthalm Plast Reconstruct Surg* 18(1):40–44 Epicanthoplasty: subcutaneous approach through ext. skin incision	*Plast Reconstruct Surg* 110(1):293–300 Med. Epicanthoplasty combined with Pilcation of Med. Canth. Tendon
Country	China (Hangzhou Zhejiang Univ. Med School)	Japan	USA	Korea (Kyungpook National Univ. Hospital)
Conjunctival suturing				
Skin incision				
Remove skin				
Orbicularis			Excise offending orbicularis underlying the epicanthal fold	
Orbital septum				
Preaponeurotic fat				
Crease form				
Suture				
Days left in				
Effectiveness				
Comments	Scanning EM showed aponeurotic fibers penetrate orbicularis to fuse with skin	Basing skin resection on whether brown position is ptotic		

continued

Modern Literature on Asian Eyelid Surgery (in English)				
Author	WM Yoo, SH Park, DR Kwang	Hwang, Kim et al	Lam, Kim	SH Chen, Mardini S, Chen HC et al
Year	2002	2003	2003	2004
Journal	*Plast Reconstruct Surg* 109(6):2067–2071 Root Z-epicanthoplasty in Asian Eyelid	*Annals of Plast Surg* 50(2):156–159	*Aesth Surg J* 23(3):170–176 Partial-incision technique	*Plast Reconstruct Surg* 114(5): 1270–1277 Corrective Asian Blepharoplasty after failed revisions
Country	Korea	Korea (Inha & Yonsei U)	USA/Korea	Taiwan (Chang Gung U)
Conjunctival suturing				
Skin incision			15–18 mm wide skin incision	
Remove skin			No	
Orbicularis			Through orbic	
Orbital septum			Open	
Preaponeurotic fat			Partial excision	
Crease form			Levator/inf. skin edge	
Suture				
Days left in				
Effectiveness				
Comments	(See JI Park's 1996 PRS article on Z-epicanthoplasty)	Lateral septoaponeurotic artery as source of bleeding during upper blepharoplasty	Clin photo shows skin incision spans $^3/_4$ of width of ciliary margin. Crease may appear deeper centrally. (See Yang's 2001 paper)	A general discussion of factors that lead to failures and its corrections

Index